The Complete
Fertility Organizer

The Complete Fertility Organizer

*A Guidebook and
Record Keeper for Women*

Manya DeLeon Miller, L.P.N., M.P.H

John Wiley & Sons, Inc.

ISBN: 978-1-62045-699-6

10   9   8   7   6   5   4   3   2   1

Contents

Foreword

P. Ronald Clisham, M.D.

When Manya Miller told me about *The Complete Fertility Organizer*, I thought, "what a clever, simple, and practical book." I asked her where I could get copies for my patients and she told me that it had yet to be written. I was so enthusiastic about her book that I wanted to help her write it. It was surprising to me that with all of the books about infertility that are currently in press, no one has thought to develop a "daytimer" for fertility patients.

Going through a fertility workup is a search for clues to the cause of a problem. Your physician will collect an incredible amount of information in a very short time about your reproductive system. Keeping this information organized will provide you with a record of where you are going and where you have been. As expensive as fertility evaluations can be, it pays to keep track of studies so they don't have to be repeated. If you ever have to change physicians, you have your own records to take with you.

The Complete Fertility Organizer is a thoughtful compilation of charts and graphs for you to use to make a record of your fertility journey. They are laid out in a problem-oriented manner to help you understand your fertility problem. Your physician may find these charts helpful since they were developed along the lines of a standard infertility evaluation. The extensive index is a valuable compilation of common scientific terms, references, and web sites used in the reproductive sciences.

Understanding your fertility problem is a major step toward its resolution. Understanding a problem allows you to participate in its solution. In this organizer, Manya Miller, with her light and effervescent dialogue, will walk you through its tables and charts to help you reach this understanding. Understanding benefits you and your physician because it allows you to work in more of a collaboration with each other through improved communication. As a physician, it's always great to know that you and your patient are on the same page in the book. As with any book, good ones are hard to put down. Here's hoping for your happy ending.

Preface

Have you been trying to get pregnant but are not pregnant yet? Are you working with an infertility specialist? Are you afraid that getting pregnant may be more of a challenge than you anticipated? Are you undergoing any treatment for infertility? If any one of these is true for you, *The Complete Fertility Organizer* is designed specifically for your needs.

The concept of fertility dwells in many contexts: the fertile ground yields plentiful food; the fertile mind yields creation; the fertile woman yields children. Fertility is an essential part of each woman's being and we are aware of it from our youngest years, whether or not we decide to have children. The realization that we might have a fertility problem—whatever the cause—can be painful, frightening, and confusing.

One wonderful thing about modern medical technology is that there is potential for nearly every woman who wants to conceive a child to do so. But enlisting that technology—taking advantage of all the available therapies—can be complex, even daunting. It can become difficult to incorporate all of the benefits that modern medicine has to offer while maintaining a sense of control.

The Complete Fertility Organizer is designed to help you organize your fertility care and help create a collaborative relationship between you and your physician. It provides mechanisms for tracking all of the information related to your infertility evaluation and treatment, including tests, monthly charts, medications, procedures, and references. When you track your own medical information, you will be responsible for an integral part of your fertility management and you will be able to provide key information to your physician. The process of organizing this information enables you to become an active participant in your own fertility care.

The Complete Fertility Organizer will be a helpful companion as you journey through infertility evaluation, treatment, and, hopefully, pregnancy.

Acknowledgments

I would like to extend my gratitude to many people for their assistance in creating this book. P. Ronald Clisham, M.D., was instrumental in this project. Enthusiasm permeated each review of the manuscript, and his contribution to the organizer's structure was tremendous. Dr. Clisham's knowledge about infertility has been an essential ingredient in making this a useful tool for women seeking pregnancy, and I am delighted to have worked with him. Jeff Braun, as well as Betsy Thorpe and the John Wiley and Sons team, were enormously helpful and supportive of this project; it is an honor to be one of their authors and to add this organizer to their excellent line of books. I deeply appreciate the contribution of my many friends and colleagues who reviewed the text and contributed helpful comments, insights, and suggestions. To my family both near and far, please accept my heartfelt thanks for your love, support, and guidance. And I would like to add my profoundest thanks to my husband: for everything.

PART ONE

Introduction

Women often spend many years dreading a positive pregnancy test, only to begin—one day, often quite unexpectedly—dreading the negative one. We shift dramatically from fearing pregnancy to wishing for it. So goes the jokingly said cliché—before the reality of the situation sets in—that one wishes for a negative pregnancy test only to later wish for a positive one, and tears result from either if it happens at the wrong time.

It's not funny, though. The cliché represents a deeper problem than can often be articulated: unwanted pregnancy can be a very serious and traumatic thing; unwanted childlessness can be equally traumatic.

Infertility, subfertility, and miscarriage are by nature isolating experiences. As women, we expect that the moment we try to have children, our fertile bodies will kick into action, become pregnant, and bear our beloved offspring into the world. When this does not happen, we may feel alone, ashamed, inadequate, guilty, angry, or a variety of unexpected emotions. The fact that even under the best of circumstances women have only about a 20 percent chance of conceiving per cycle does little to steer us away from the idea that our success at childbearing is virtually insured.

A couple may seek some type of assistance after they have unsuccessfully tried to get pregnant for a period of time: they may consult medical books; the woman might pay a visit to her gynecologist or an infertility specialist; the man might obtain a urological consult. They might ask the advice of friends who have had similar experiences. Perhaps the couple will continue trying on their own, using information gleaned from these various resources, and keep hoping that something will work.

Often something will work. If the couple has no significant obstacles to fertility, or if the problem is only in gauging the most fertile time of the month, these approaches will usually remove the hurdle to bearing a child. In fact, most of the time there is nothing wrong with the couple at all, and it is just a matter of letting the 20 percent success rate per cycle kick in. After a year of trying to conceive, about 85 percent of couples will be pregnant. Within two years, about 95 percent will be pregnant. This is a very happy ending.

Sometimes, though, the going is a little tougher. The solutions—indeed, the problems themselves—may be more complex. Medical assistance may be required. A complete infertility evaluation may be necessary. Treatments may be required. The journey may be rough at times, but the goal—a child—is worthy of the couple's efforts.

Each couple is unique, and what each has to face is unique as well. Despite the similarities among popular medical references regarding infertility (after reading two or three, they seem woefully repetitive), the diagnosis and treatment for a particular couple is singular—as singular as the couple itself. The path to motherhood, decorated along the way with thrills and melancholy, cannot be documented by others—it can only be documented by those individuals themselves marching upon it. Take 100 women who delivered infants and you will have 100 glorious stories of childbirth; take 100 women striving for fertility and you will have 100 stories of how they are attempting motherhood. *The Complete Fertility Organizer* is for *your* story, designed to provide a place for all of the medical information related to *your* infertility evaluation, treatment, and pregnancy.

HOW THIS BOOK EVOLVED—THE AUTHOR'S PERSPECTIVE After trying to become pregnant without assistance other than that of an ordinary gynecologist and the reference books I read so fervently, my husband and I were elated when I became pregnant. After what seemed like an eternity, we were to be parents at last! The thought of a problem was inconceivable, though I found out later that those with prior difficulty getting pregnant are more likely (for many and diverse reasons) to endure problems later on such as miscarriage or pre-term birth. At eight weeks, I miscarried. Dedicated as we were, despite our sadness, we kept trying, and three months later I found myself in the hospital with a ruptured ectopic pregnancy. But again, upon my recovery, we kept trying, this time seeking better medical help from an infertility specialist.

And it is this last experience that serves as the motivation for this organizer. While witnessing all that medical technology has to offer, I feel the need to keep track of my own key medical information; keeping track of things allows me to be an active participant in my own care. Reproductive endocrinology and the science of infertility are rapidly blossoming fields that benefit from the expertise of caring and devoted health care professionals as well as research, which contributes to increased knowledge at a heady pace. But the highly technical and rapidly advancing nature of this field can be confusing; it is easy to misunderstand procedures, terminology, and treatments. Although plenty of books provide technical information about infertility evaluation and treatment, they are general in scope: they do not focus on each person's specific obstacles to fertility. Our own problems quickly become lost in books that discuss all possible problems. In a sea of infertility information, our own issues can nearly drown, and our methods for coping often drown along with them. So, too, can our ability to see solutions and find the strength to weather the process. In addition, these feelings can prevent us from developing a good rapport with our infertility specialist.

This organizer is different because it focuses on *you* and *your fertility;* it allows you to track your information and profile your fertility situation. When you use this organizer, you will feel more secure about where you are in the fertility process, what your unique obstacles are, what your goal is, and what steps you have taken toward that goal.

KEEPING TRACK OF THINGS—HOW TO USE THIS ORGANIZER The objective of this journal is to be a companion along your road to having a baby—to work in concert with other references, resources, and your physician. As with most things done well, keeping a record of your efforts is a good idea. If you use the charts and tables in this organizer, you will have a clear picture of where you've been and where you're going, helping you to communicate with your physician along the way. Most of the writing in this book will be yours: the medical wisdom housed in other books will not be repeated. This organizer is not intended to replace the advice of your physician: it is intended to facilitate a collaboration with your physician, allowing you to get the most out of your infertility treatment.

Since it is frequently the woman who initiates infertility treatment, this book is geared toward her, though not to the exclusion of the male, who has record-keeping sections, too. Either partner may complete the sections in this book. In fact, there is no prescribed way to use this book: it may be completed in whatever way is most useful for you. If the narrative contains things you already know about fertility, please do not feel constrained by the text; simply skip to the charts and use them as you wish. Just as the path to parenthood will be unique for each person, so, too, will be the use of this book. It is perfectly fine to skip any sections you do not need right now, and it is fine to start using this organizer before you have seen an infertility specialist. But when you do go visit your physician, take this organizer with you to your appointments, since having it with you will encourage collaboration with your physician and the information within it will assist him or her enormously. Also, having the organizer with you gives you a place to document information that comes up during the appointment for future reference.

The Complete Fertility Organizer charts are presented in three sections: the Charts About You section tracks information about your baseline infertility evaluation. It includes information about your medical history, initial infertility tests, monthly cycles, treatments, and other useful information. The Charts About Information section tracks references, questions you have and answers you receive, and financial information. The Once You Are Pregnant section is available to track information related to your healthy pregnancy once you become pregnant.

A listing of resources—books, journals, organizations, and web sites—is included to help you find comprehensive fertility information. Also included is a glossary of key terms related to fertility; the glossary expands on some concepts not covered elsewhere in the text.

PART TWO

Charts about You

Your Infertility Evaluation

This first chart is a place for you to track the results of your initial infertility evaluation. There is room for many diagnostic test results. You probably will not need all of them; feel free to leave those you do not need blank. The goal of this chart is for you to have, at your fingertips, the results of your initial infertility evaluations. Having the results readily available will make it easier for you to understand your situation, and will encourage a collaborative relationship with your physician. Also, if you decide to go to a new physician at some point, the chart will provide pertinent medical information until your physician can see your previous medical records. This chart covers five major areas of fertility: ovulation, fallopian tubes/pelvic factors, male factor, cervical factor, and sexuality. These five areas are the same ones that most infertility specialists will evaluate; since you will be conceptualizing of fertility in a similar way, your relationship with your physician will be enhanced and communication will be improved. As you work arm-in-arm with your physician to chart results from your evaluations, your understanding of your own fertility issues will increase dramatically.

Before going on to the charts, let's examine five major areas of infertility evaluation and some of the tools your physician might use to evaluate you:

OVULATION Each month, a woman's reproductive system undergoes a complex cycle to prepare for pregnancy. Though preparation for pregnancy actually begins a few days before her menstrual period begins, day one of the cycle is considered the day the woman's menstrual period starts. During her period, the lining of her uterus is shed in response to falling hormone levels from the prior month's cycle. The pituitary gland—a small endocrine gland in the brain—releases hormones into the bloodstream. One of the hormones—follicle-stimulating hormone (FSH)—begins to recruit (or develop) follicles in the ovaries. Follicles are round, fluid-filled compartments, each containing an egg, and the FSH helps them grow and mature. As they grow, these follicles produce estrogen. Estrogen makes the uterine lining thick and receptive to embryo implantation later on. The increasing estrogen level also allows glands near the cervix (the opening into the uterus) to release thin, stretchy, clear mucus. This mucus helps sperm enter the uterus through the cervix.

When the estrogen level reaches a peak, the pituitary gland releases a hormone called luteinizing hormone (LH) into the bloodstream. The LH is released in a surge, which signals important genetic divisions to take place in the egg; these divisions mature the egg so that it can be fertilized. The LH surge also causes the follicle to rupture. Ovulation (the release of the egg) takes place about 34 to 36 hours after the beginning of the LH surge.

After the egg is released, the follicle transforms itself into what is called the corpus luteum, which produces and releases the hormone progesterone. Progesterone makes the uterine lining soft, nutritive, and able to support a pregnancy. It also causes the cervical mucus to thicken and behave like a barrier to the uterus. (This is exactly opposite of what the estrogen did around the time of ovulation!) Unless directed otherwise, the corpus luteum will last for 9 to 11 days before it begins to regress (or shrink); when it regresses, the estrogen and progesterone levels drop, the uterine lining sheds, the menstrual period begins—and the whole cycle starts again.

If, however, an egg is fertilized by a sperm, the resulting embryo will implant into the soft uterine lining and begin producing a hormone called human chorionic gonadotropin (hCG). The hCG signals the corpus luteum that progesterone and estrogen are still required, so that it will not regress. These hormones maintain the embryo (and make sure the uterine lining is not shed) until the placenta can take over hormone production.

During your infertility evaluation, one of the first things your physician might want to explore is whether you are ovulating. Here are some of the tools your physician might use to see if you are ovulating:

1. Basal body temperature monitoring. One thing you can do to see if you are ovulating is take your temperature daily; this is called basal body temperature (BBT) monitoring. You will take your temperature before getting out of bed each morning and then chart your temperature on a graph. If charted carefully, BBT monitoring suggests when you are ovulating. Why does it work? One of progesterone's effects is that it increases body temperature a half to a whole degree; if you chart your BBT each day, you can see this temperature increase after you have ovulated. Your temperature will usually stay at the elevated level for at least 11 days after ovulation. If you do not become pregnant, the corpus luteum will cease functioning, the progesterone levels will fall, and your temperature will drop to pre-ovulation levels. Of course, this low-tech approach is not perfect: it can sometimes be inaccurate (for instance, if you have a fever it might look like you ovulated when you did not) and it can become rather stressful at times (taking your temperature daily and waiting to retrospectively learn if you've ovulated can become difficult; if this should happen to you, talk with your physician). However, BBT monitoring is a useful method that can reveal a lot about your cycle, and it is an inexpensive means of assessing ovulation on your own.

HOW TO MONITOR YOUR BASAL BODY TEMPERATURE

Basal body temperature monitoring is simple and inexpensive to perform. All you will need is a thermometer (glass mercury, digital, or special basal body thermometer all work fine, though the latter is easier to read and may be more precise) and a pen or a pencil. Set the thermometer by your bedside before you go to sleep and when you first wake up—before you drink anything, eat anything, smoke anything, walk anywhere, brush your teeth, or exercise—take your temperature. (Any activity, no matter how slight, can increase your temperature and give you a misleading result. If you are using a glass thermometer, shake it down before going to sleep—even that movement can increase your temperature!) After you get a reading, chart it immediately (waiting is not good, especially if you are sleepy, because you may forget what your temperature was). Do this every day. Once you have a cycle charted, you should see a pattern: your temperature will probably be about a half to a whole degree higher in the second half of your cycle than in the first. The day that corresponds to the initial increase in temperature will usually be about a day or two after you have ovulated. Remember: the temperature increases under the influence of progesterone, which comes from the corpus luteum after ovulation. Do not wait until after the increase to have intercourse because by then you will have missed ovulation! BBT charting is useful for several reasons even though it gives us only retrospective information about when ovulation occurred. A BBT chart can indicate a lot about your hormones and ovulation, and may be helpful to the infertility specialist in evaluating you. Also, if your cycles are fairly regular, you may be able to use one month's chart to predict when you will ovulate the next month, and have intercourse accordingly.

2. Cervical mucus monitoring. As estrogen increases during the first half of the menstrual cycle, cervical mucus production increases, too. Around the time of ovulation, the increasing estrogen makes the mucus at the entry to the cervix stretchy, springy, crystal clear, and copious—just right to help the sperm gain entry into the uterus. (I had a nurse practitioner who called cervical mucus "highways for sperm"—I've always liked that term!) Keeping track of the quality of your cervical mucus can indicate when ovulation is about to take place.

HOW TO MONITOR YOUR CERVICAL MUCUS

There are many excellent resources available (see the References and Resources section for some) that give great detail about cervical mucus monitoring and fertility signals; they are well worth reading. This is only a brief introduction to cervical mucus monitoring to get you started.

As we discussed earlier, as estrogen levels increase during the first half of the menstrual cycle, the cervical mucus changes: it becomes optically clear, stretchy, springy, and plentiful. It almost looks like raw egg white. This is in contrast to the tacky, opaque, or sparse mucus that is usually present. When the mucus begins changing, it is a sign that your estrogen levels are increasing and ovulation is approaching. You can check your cervical mucus using your fingers by gently inserting them into your vagina each day at about the same time (prior to sexual activity, which can make it difficult to correctly assess the mucus) and feeling its consistency. The mucus is released from around the cervix into the vagina and you will be able to feel it with your fingers. Is it slippery? Can a strand stay intact when pulled between two fingers? Is it clear? Is it copious? As these qualities become apparent, ovulation generally is nearing. Tracking the quality of your cervical mucus gives you a clue about when you will ovulate. One nice thing about this type of monitoring is that the cervical mucus changes before ovulation and not after, so you can anticipate ovulation and time intercourse.

It is perfectly all right if you do not feel comfortable using your fingers to check your cervical mucus. Many women can feel the increased mid-cycle wetness of the vagina or feel the slippery consistency of the cervical mucus on tissue without checking directly. No matter which way you decide to monitor this fertility sign, you can keep track of which days have heightened cervical mucus on the sympto-thermal tracking chart in the Charts about You section.

3. Ovulation predictor kits. A little earlier we discussed how ovulation takes place after the LH surge. Ovulation predictor kits work by detecting

LH presence in the urine. Your physician will tell you when in your cycle to start testing; then, at the same time each day, you will test your urine. When the color of the test stripe or dot is darker than the control stripe or dot, it means you are having your LH surge. When the LH surge occurs, you know that you will ovulate within approximately 24 to 36 hours. Two nice things about ovulation predictor kits are that they are used in the privacy of your own home and they give reliable information about the timing of your ovulation before it occurs. Ovulation predictor kits can be purchased at many drug stores and by mail. Your physician may have a preferred brand of test kit—be sure to ask.

4. Progesterone measurement. As mentioned earlier, progesterone levels increase during the second half of the cycle. Since the corpus luteum is responsible for this increase (and the corpus luteum comes into being only after ovulation), an increased level of progesterone lets you know that ovulation has taken place. A blood sample in the second half of your cycle allows measurement of the circulating progesterone; a level of 10 ng/mL or higher suggests that ovulation occurred.

5. Ultrasound. Ultrasonography uses high-frequency sound waves to create an image of internal tissues without the danger of x-rays or radiation. In a transvaginal ultrasound, a wand shaped device is inserted into the vagina and the sound waves create a picture on a screen, detailed enough to reveal the follicles in the ovaries. Developing follicles grow at a very steady pace: about 2 mm per day. They naturally release their eggs when they are about 20 mm (a little less than an inch) in diameter. (In a clomiphene stimulated cycle, they release their eggs when they are about 24 mm in diameter.) This is very helpful! If your physician sees that your follicle is 16 mm on Monday, he will know that on Tuesday it will be 18 mm, and on Thursday it will be 20 mm—ready to release the egg. Ultrasound can assess how well your

hormones have prepared your uterine lining (the endometrium) by measuring the thickness of the lining; they can also check for cysts on your ovaries or other factors that may be affecting your fertility. Ultrasound is an excellent method of finding out about your cycle, and can pinpoint almost exactly when you will ovulate.

These are basic tools used to determine if you are ovulating and assess any difficulty you may be having with your ovulation. Later on, if you decide to have any infertility treatments, these tools may be used again to precisely time procedures (such as artificial insemination) with your ovulation. Other evaluations are available, if you need them, such as endometrial biopsy or other types of tests. To keep track of information about your ovulation, there is a supply of Your Detailed Monthly Charts later in this section. They allow you to chart your BBT, cervical mucus, ovulation predictor kits, ultrasound results, and hormone levels all in one place, making your hormonal complexities simpler to understand.

FALLOPIAN TUBES/PELVIC FACTORS Fallopian tubes are the thin tubes extending from the left and right sides of the uterus toward the left and right ovaries. At the ends of the fallopian tubes are delicate petals called fimbria. These fimbria do not connect with the ovaries, but, at the time of ovulation, they coax the egg off of the surface of the ovary and into the funnel-shaped ampullary portion of the fallopian tube. The sperm will have traveled from the vagina through the cervix, up through the uterus, and up the fallopian tube, where one will fertilize the egg in the fallopian tube. Once the sperm and the egg have united their genetic material, the cells begin dividing and growing, slowly moving down the fallopian tube into the uterus. It takes about three days for the embryo to reach the uterus, after which it implants in the rich uterine lining.

It is easy to see why having patent (open) fallopian tubes is so important! The sperm need to travel up unobstructed tubes to get to the egg, and the embryo needs to travel down an unobstructed tube to get to the uterus. Anything that blocks the tubes or makes them rough can prevent conception. Also, the fimbria need to be able to move freely enough to coax the egg off of the ovary; if the fimbria are stuck together for some reason, the egg will not make it into the fallopian tube where the sperm are waiting.

There are several things that can interfere with fallopian tube functioning. Infections (like sexually transmitted infections) can make the delicate lining of the fallopian tubes scarred and rough; scar tissue can block the tubes or can prevent the fimbria from picking up the egg. Endometriosis is a condition in which some of the uterine lining finds its way out of the uterus and into the pelvic region. The lining can implant outside of the uterus and cause adhesions on and scarring of the fallopian tubes or other organs. Some of the symptoms of adhesions and scarring are pain with intercourse, severe pain with menstruation, and pelvic pain. Sometimes, however, there are no symptoms at all.

Sometimes a woman's uterus, ovaries, or fallopian tubes may have formed abnormally, and her anatomy may not be conducive to conceiving or carrying a baby. Such congenital abnormalities may range from mild to severe, and are quite rare. Or, a woman may have had surgery that can interfere with conception or pregnancy.

Here are some of the tools your physician might use to assess your fallopian tubes and pelvic region:

1. Hysterosalpingogram (HSG). To view the structure of your uterus, fallopian tubes, ovaries, and pelvic region, a special x-ray is taken a week to ten days after the beginning of your period. This test is done prior to ovulation to avoid flushing out an embryo or exposing an embryo to x-rays. A very thin tube is inserted into your cervix and a dye is injected. The dye flows through your uterus, up your fallopian tubes, and, if the tubes are

open, spills out into your abdominal cavity. X-rays are taken as the dye works its way through the tubes and into the abdomen. These x-rays outline your tubes and uterus; if the fluid cannot pass through the tube, blockages or abnormalities may be present. The HSG is a very useful test, and reveals a lot about your reproductive organs. It may also be therapeutic: your fertility may actually be enhanced! The dilation of the fallopian tubes during the exam and the use of certain dyes may increase your chances for pregnancy during the three months after the exam.

2. Laparoscopy. If your HSG suggests a problem or your physician thinks additional investigation is necessary, you may have a laparoscopy performed. A laparoscopy is a surgical procedure in which a laparoscope (a small fiberoptic device) is inserted into your abdomen while you are under anesthesia. This device allows your physician to examine your pelvic organs and see if there is scar tissue, adhesions, abnormalities, or endometriosis. This procedure can detect more subtle problems than an HSG can. In fact, some problems may actually be surgically corrected during the laparoscopy procedure.

3. Tests for infection. Your physician may order tests to see if you are or have ever been infected with sexually transmitted infections that can result in scarring or adhesions of your fallopian tubes and ovaries. For example, a culture for chlamydia may be performed by swabbing your cervix and seeing if the bacteria grow in a culture medium, revealing the presence of an infection. Or a blood test might be done to measure anti-chlamydia antibodies, components of the immune system that signal past exposure to chlamydia.

MALE FACTOR Sperm are produced by the millions in the male's testicles. Sperm begin to develop in the seminiferous tubules in each testicle;

interspersed among the developing sperm are testosterone-producing Leydig cells. It takes about 70 to 72 days for sperm formation; once formed, the sperm leave the seminiferous tubules and move through the rete testis into the epididymis. It takes the sperm an additional 12 to 21 days to move through the epididymis and be prepared for ejaculation, during which time a maturation process takes place. Once mature and capable of swimming, the sperm travel through the vas deferens and are joined by fluids from the seminal vesicles and the prostate gland; the resulting fluid is called semen and is released upon ejaculation. Of the millions of sperm in the semen, just one will ultimately fertilize the waiting egg.

As much as 40 percent of infertility is thought to be related to male factor issues. These include problems with the sperm, the semen, male hormone production, anatomy, and function.

There are a variety of tests available to assess male fertility problems; however, the basic study undertaken to evaluate male factor fertility is a semen analysis. A semen analysis reveals a lot of information about male fertility. The male will be asked to abstain from ejaculation for a specified period of time (usually two or three days) and then give a semen sample. This sample will be analyzed under a high-power microscope. The number of sperm will be counted, and their movement ability (motility) and shape (morphology) observed. Sperm can be normal in one way, but abnormal in another. For instance, there might be a normal number of sperm, but the shape may be abnormal. Or there might be a smaller number of normally shaped sperm. Each pattern might be a clue to a specific diagnosis. Signs of infection—like the presence of white blood cells in the semen—will be explored, too. If the sperm or semen is not normal, it might be a clue to the problem at hand. Some reasons for abnormal sperm or semen include testicular heat, exposure to medications, illness, infection, or structural abnormalities.

Generally, more than one semen sample over a period of weeks or months will be requested. Why? Sperm measured today reflect what was happening in the male approximately 90 days ago. If the male had an infection that has since resolved, or if he was under stress or taking medication, the older sperm might look abnormal but the newer sperm may be perfectly fine. Also, sometimes abnormalities are transient and can resolve spontaneously on their own. Usually only a persistent pattern of abnormality over several analyses is cause for concern.

CERVICAL FACTOR The cervix is the portal of entry through which the sperm travel to reach the uterus, the fallopian tubes, and, finally, the egg. Usually, the cervix is tightly closed and there is thick mucus blocking entry of bacteria and viruses into the sterile uterus. However, as mentioned earlier, prior to ovulation this mucus changes: it becomes thin, clear, stretchy, and very accommodating to sperm. The cervical mucus is secreted by cervical glands in response to estrogen. The mucus behaves rather like a gatekeeper, allowing the sperm to enter the uterus in a slow, steady stream. (If the cervical mucus were not there, the sperm could rush into the uterus all at once. An egg would have to be in the fallopian tubes waiting or a chance for conception could be easily missed. The reservoir of sperm in the cervical mucus increases the window of opportunity for conception.) If there is not enough mucus to help the sperm gain entry to the uterus, or it is too thick or is abnormal in some way, fertility can be impaired.

Some of the tools used to evaluate cervical factors include:

1. Post-coital test (also called PCT or Huhners' Test). This test is usually performed around the time of ovulation, when your cervical mucus production is at its peak. You and your partner will be asked to have intercourse a specific number of hours before the test is scheduled (your physician will help you time this correctly). Afterwards, your physician will remove a small quantity of your cervical mucus. First, the mucus will be examined to see if it is the right quantity (copious), if it is stretchy

(spinnbarkeit), and if it ferns (a response to estrogen that makes the mucus fern-shaped when dried on a microscopic slide). Then it will be examined under a powerful microscope. There should be some visible sperm moving in the cervical mucus, even hours after intercourse. If there are not, this may be a clue that something is the matter with the sperm-mucus interaction. If the sperm appear abnormal within your mucus, your physician may refer your partner for semen analysis. If you do not have enough mucus or it is too thick (this is sometimes called "hostile cervical mucus"), there are various procedures available to overcome this barrier to fertility.

2. Physical exam. Inflammation or infection of the cervix can cause the cervical mucus to be an inappropriate environment for the sperm. Sometimes an inflamed cervix is visible upon exam; the cervix may also be swabbed and cultured to see if there is an infection. If an infection is found, antibiotics might be given, and the cervical environment given a chance to return to normal.

3. Medical history review. Sometimes information from your medical history can reveal a clue to a fertility problem. A Pap smear is a test for the early detection of cancer; it works by taking a swab of cells from the cervix and then looking for abnormal, precancerous cells under a microscope. If a woman has had an abnormal Pap smear, she may also have had a procedure such as cautery, freezing, or biopsy to remove and further test the abnormal tissue. Sometimes this process can damage the cervix and the mucus-producing glands. This can lead to inadequate cervical mucus production. One way of overcoming this problem is with intrauterine insemination (IUI), a procedure in which prepared sperm are inserted directly into the uterus through a tube, bypassing the cervix altogether.

SEXUALITY Sexuality is an important, indeed essential, facet of fertility. Not only is sexuality an integral factor in becoming pregnant, information about sexuality can yield clues to a fertility problem. Your physician may ask about the sexual relationship between you and your partner. Here are some of the questions you might be asked, along with the reasons:

1. How frequently do you have intercourse? When do you have intercourse? Are you aware of when you are ovulating? Do you have intercourse when you are ovulating?

2. Do you have pain with intercourse? Pain during sexual relations can be the result of scarring, adhesions, endometriosis, or other problems affecting the pelvic region. This clue can lead to a diagnosis.

3. Do you use lubricants? Even water-based lubricants can be rather effective as contraceptives, hindering pregnancy rather than assisting it. Your physician may recommend other practices if you are having difficulty with inadequate lubrication.

4. Do you get right up after sex? If after every lovemaking session you jump right out of bed and run to the restroom, many of the sperm, due to the force of gravity, may not have a chance to enter the uterus.

Your physician may ask you other questions, too. You might feel comfortable discussing these intimate matters, but if you do not, let your physician know. He or she might be able to ask fewer questions, ask only a few at a time, or prepare a list that you can answer at home in writing.

The first chart in this section allows you to track the basic evaluations we have just discussed, plus others you may have performed during your initial infertility evaluation. Monitoring your basal body temperature, cervical mucus, and ovulation predictor kit use may play a big role in your infertility evaluation and can be charted on Your Detailed Monthly Charts. There are many other diagnostic evaluations available, depending on your situation and circumstances, but they are not routine for everyone. For additional information, consult the resources listed at the end of the organizer; they can explain the available diagnostic tools in wonderful detail. For each test you undergo, ask your physician what the results mean in your case and write down any extra information about the results that might help you remember it and understand it in the future.

Ovulation

Test	Date	Results/Comments
ultrasound		day in cycle
❏ abdominal		date expect ovulation
❏ transvaginal		
		right ovary
		number follicles
		dimensions (mm)
		left ovary
		number follicles
		dimensions (mm)
endometrial biopsy		day in cycle
		interpretation

Comments

Blood Tests

Test	Date	Results (units)	Day in Menstrual Cycle	Normal Range	Interpretation
androstenedione					
DHEAS					
estradiol					
free T3					
free testosterone					
free thyroxine (T4)					
FSH					
glucose					
insulin					
LH					
LH to FSH ratio					
progesterone					
prolactin					
thyroid-stimulating hormone					
17-hydroxyprogesterone					
total testosterone					
other					
other					
other					
other					
other					

Comments

Fallopian Tubes/Pelvic Factor

Test	Date	Results/Comments
hysterosalpingogram		
		uterine shape: ❑ normal ❑ abnormal
		if abnormal, type of abnormality
		fallopian tubal patency: right
		left other
laparoscopy		endometriosis ❑ yes ❑ no
		if yes, stage
		location
		adhesions ❑ yes ❑ no
		if yes, location
		fallopian tubal patency: right
		left other
hysteroscopy		endometriosis ❑ yes ❑ no
		if yes, stage
		location
		adhesions ❑ yes ❑ no
		if yes, location
		fallopian tubal patency: right
		left other
falloposcopy		endometriosis ❑ yes ❑ no
		if yes, stage
		location
		adhesions ❑ yes ❑ no
		if yes, location
		fallopian tubal patency: right
		left other

Comments

Tests for Infections Past and Present

Test	Date	Type (e.g., blood, cervical swab, etc)	Result	Interpretation
chlamydia			❏ positive ❏ negative	
			❏ past ❏ current	
cytomegalovirus			❏ positive ❏ negative	
			❏ past ❏ current	
hepatitis (specify type)			❏ positive ❏ negative	
			❏ past ❏ current	
herpes virus II			❏ positive ❏ negative	
			❏ currently active	
HIV			❏ positive ❏ negative	
mycoplasma			❏ positive ❏ negative	
			❏ past ❏ current	
rubella			❏ positive ❏ negative	
			❏ past ❏ current	
syphilis			❏ positive ❏ negative	
			❏ past ❏ current	
toxoplasmosis			❏ positive ❏ negative	
			❏ past ❏ current	
other			❏ positive ❏ negative	
			❏ past ❏ current	
other			❏ positive ❏ negative	
			❏ past ❏ current	
other			❏ positive ❏ negative	
			❏ past ❏ current	
other			❏ positive ❏ negative	
			❏ past ❏ current	

Male Factor

Test	Date	Results/Comments	
semen analysis #1		volume (cc)	sperm count
		motility	morphology
		round cells present? ❑ yes ❑ no	
		comments	
semen analysis #2		volume (cc)	sperm count
		motility	morphology
		round cells present? ❑ yes ❑ no	
		comments	
semen analysis #3		volume (cc)	sperm count
		motility	morphology
		round cells present? ❑ yes ❑ no	
		comments	
semen analysis #4		volume (cc)	sperm count
		motility	morphology
		round cells present? ❑ yes ❑ no	
physical exam		comments	
urinalysis		❑ normal ❑ abnormal ❑ indeterminate	
testicular ultrasound		❑ normal ❑ abnormal ❑ indeterminate	
testicular biopsy		❑ normal ❑ abnormal ❑ indeterminate	
vasography		❑ normal ❑ abnormal ❑ indeterminate	
other test		value	
		interpretation	
other test		value	
		interpretation	
other test		value	
		interpretation	

Tests for Infections Past and Present (Male Factor)

Test	Date	Type (e.g., blood, cervical swab, etc)	Result		Interpretation
chlamydia			❑ positive	❑ negative	
			❑ past	❑ current	
cytomegalovirus			❑ positive	❑ negative	
			❑ past	❑ current	
hepatitis (specify type)			❑ positive	❑ negative	
			❑ past	❑ current	
herpes virus II			❑ positive	❑ negative	
			❑ currently active		
HIV			❑ positive	❑ negative	
mycoplasma			❑ positive	❑ negative	
			❑ past	❑ current	
rubella			❑ positive	❑ negative	
			❑ past	❑ current	
syphilis			❑ positive	❑ negative	
			❑ past	❑ current	
toxoplasmosis			❑ positive	❑ negative	
			❑ past	❑ current	
other			❑ positive	❑ negative	
			❑ past	❑ current	
other			❑ positive	❑ negative	
			❑ past	❑ current	
other			❑ positive	❑ negative	
			❑ past	❑ current	
other			❑ positive	❑ negative	
			❑ past	❑ current	

Cervical Factor

Test	Date	Results/Comments
post-coital test		mucus amount ___ spinnbarkeit ___
		ferning ___ viscosity ___
		number of sperm visualized ___ per ___
		comments ___
		___
		day in cycle ___
		❏ normal ❏ abnormal ❏ indeterminate
physical evaluation of cervix		interpretation ___
		___
Pap smear		❏ within normal limits ❏ abnormal cells
		describe ___
		___
other test		value ___
		interpretation ___
other test		value ___
		interpretation ___
other test		value ___
		interpretation ___
other test		value ___
		interpretation ___

Comments

_____

_____

_____

_____

_____

_____

Sexuality

Subject	Date	Results/Comments
Pain with intercourse?		❑ yes ❑ no
		If yes, when did it start?
		Is it all the time?
		Where is it?
Frequency of intercourse		times/week
		Any unusual schedules (e.g., work)?
Lubricants used?		❑ yes ❑ no ❑ sometimes
		if yes, what type?
Other questions or		
concerns about		
sexuality and fertility:		

Comments

Other Tests That Might Be Performed (Female)

Test	Date	Results/Comments
weight		❑ pounds ❑ kilograms
height		❑ inches ❑ centimeters
blood pressure		/ mm Hg
		❑ right arm ❑ left arm
		❑ lying ❑ sitting ❑ standing
blood type		❑ A ❑ B ❑ O ❑ AB
		❑ Rh+ ❑ Rh-
urinalysis		❑ normal ❑ abnormal ❑ indeterminate
		interpretation
antisperm antibodies		titers IgA IgG IgM
		method
		interpretation
other test		value
		interpretation
other test		value
		interpretation
other test		value
		interpretation
other test		value
		interpretation

Comments

_____

_____

_____

_____

_____

_____

_____

Other Tests That Might Be Performed (Male)

Test	Date	Results/Comments
weight		❏ pounds ❏ kilograms
height		❏ inches ❏ centimeters
blood pressure		/ mm Hg
		❏ right arm ❏ left arm
		❏ lying ❏ sitting ❏ standing
blood type		❏ A ❏ B ❏ O ❏ AB
		❏ Rh+ ❏ Rh-
urinalysis		❏ normal ❏ abnormal ❏ indeterminate
		interpretation
antisperm antibodies		titers IgA IgG IgM
		method
		interpretation
other test		value
		interpretation
other test		value
		interpretation
other test		value
		interpretation
other test		value
		interpretation

Comments

Your Detailed Monthly Charts

I detest the small papers that I for so long collected to keep track of basal body temperatures, cervical mucus, and other information about my cycle: a batch of dog-eared, blurry graphs stapled together and, despite much care and regard, always at least a little bit crumpled. Each chart housed a jumble of temperatures, symptoms, and other information, which, after a month passed, would be absolutely illegible and uninterpretable. Checks, circles, arrows—endless symbols that blended together to mean nothing in the end! This section has clearly laid out charts for all of the key events that you might wish to track. There are plenty of charts so you can record many cycles worth of sympto-thermal information, hormone levels, ultrasound results, and more, cleanly and all in one place. Some of the information you may not wish or need to track; just track what is relevant for you. At the end of each cycle, transfer key events—like ovulation or procedures—onto the calendar in the next section. You can start using these charts even before you have your first visit with an infertility specialist; in fact, having a cycle's worth of information may be very useful to have on hand at your first visit.

Sample

Month *January* **Year** *1999*

Day Jan 4 5 6 7 8 9 10

Cycle Day	1	2	3	4	5	6	7	8	9	10	11	12	13	14	15	16	17	18	19	20	21	22	23	24	25	26	27	28	29	30	31
cervical mucus		*	*	*	*			✔				↓	↑	↑	↑	↑	↑	↓													
menstrual period																															
conception attempts								✔				✔	✔	✔			✔	✔		✔					✔		✔				
ovulation predictor kit													✔																		
follicle size by ultrasound (mm)	*no ultrasound this month*																														

Oral Temperature °F

Cycle Day	1	2	3	4	5	6	7	8	9	10	11	12	13	14	15	16	17	18	19	20	21	22	23	24	25	26	27	28	29	30	31
99.8																															
99.6																															
99.4																															
99.2																															
99.0																								●							
98.8																					●	●	●		●		●	●			
98.6																●	●	●		●			●		●	●					
98.4														●		●			●									●			
98.2													●																●		
98.0											●	●																			●
97.8									●	●																					
97.6					●		●	●																							
97.4		●		●		●		●																							
97.2			●																												
97.0																															
96.8																															

Date of ovulation *January 16, 1999* Transfer to the calendar section starting on page 57 for easy reference about the whole month.

Symbols:

↑ ovulatory mucus: slippery, copious, stretchy, clear ↓ normal mucus: dry, pasty, thick, crumbly ↑ unable to determine

* days with menstrual bleeding ✔ intercourse, artificial inseminations, assisted reproductive procedures

Information from physician: Ultrasound—follicle measurement (in mm) R = right ovary L = left ovary; Ovulation predictor kit: ✔ day of LH surge

Month _____ Year _____

Day

Cycle Day	1	2	3	4	5	6	7	8	9	10	11	12	13	14	15	16	17	18	19	20	21	22	23	24	25	26	27	28	29	30	31
cervical mucus																															
menstrual period																															
conception attempts																															
ovulation predictor kit																															
follicle size by ultrasound (mm)																															

Oral Temperature °F

Cycle Day	1	2	3	4	5	6	7	8	9	10	11	12	13	14	15	16	17	18	19	20	21	22	23	24	25	26	27	28	29	30	31
99.8																															
99.6																															
99.4																															
99.2																															
99.0																															
98.8																															
98.6																															
98.4																															
98.2																															
98.0																															
97.8																															
97.6																															
97.4																															
97.2																															
97.0																															
96.8																															

Date of ovulation _____ Transfer to the calendar section starting on page 57 for easy reference about the whole month.

Symbols:

↑ ovulatory mucus: slippery, copious, stretchy, clear ↓ normal mucus: dry, pasty, thick, crumbly → unable to determine

✱ days with menstrual bleeding ✔ intercourse, artificial inseminations, assisted reproductive procedures

Information from physician: Ultrasound—follicle measurement (in mm) R = right ovary L = left ovary; Ovulation predictor kit: ✔ day of LH surge

Month _____ Year _____

Day

Cycle Day	1	2	3	4	5	6	7	8	9	10	11	12	13	14	15	16	17	18	19	20	21	22	23	24	25	26	27	28	29	30	31
cervical mucus																															
menstrual period																															
conception attempts																															
ovulation predictor kit																															
follicle size by ultrasound (mm)																															

Oral Temperature °F

Cycle Day	1	2	3	4	5	6	7	8	9	10	11	12	13	14	15	16	17	18	19	20	21	22	23	24	25	26	27	28	29	30	31
99.8																															
99.6																															
99.4																															
99.2																															
99.0																															
98.8																															
98.6																															
98.4																															
98.2																															
98.0																															
97.8																															
97.6																															
97.4																															
97.2																															
97.0																															
96.8																															

Date of ovulation _____ Transfer to the calendar section starting on page 57 for easy reference about the whole month.

Symbols:

↑ ovulatory mucus: slippery, copious, stretchy, clear   ↓ normal mucus: dry, pasty, thick, crumbly   ↱ unable to determine

✱ days with menstrual bleeding   ✔ intercourse, artificial inseminations, assisted reproductive procedures

Information from physician: Ultrasound—follicle measurement (in mm) R = right ovary L = left ovary; Ovulation predictor kit: ✔ day of LH surge

Month _____ Year _____

Day

Cycle Day	1	2	3	4	5	6	7	8	9	10	11	12	13	14	15	16	17	18	19	20	21	22	23	24	25	26	27	28	29	30	31
cervical mucus																															
menstrual period																															
conception attempts																															
ovulation predictor kit																															
follicle size by ultrasound (mm)																															

Oral Temperature °F

Cycle Day	1	2	3	4	5	6	7	8	9	10	11	12	13	14	15	16	17	18	19	20	21	22	23	24	25	26	27	28	29	30	31
99.8																															
99.6																															
99.4																															
99.2																															
99.0																															
98.8																															
98.6																															
98.4																															
98.2																															
98.0																															
97.8																															
97.6																															
97.4																															
97.2																															
97.0																															
96.8																															

Date of ovulation _____

Transfer to the calendar section starting on page 57 for easy reference about the whole month.

Symbols:

↑ ovulatory mucus: slippery, copious, stretchy, clear   ↓ normal mucus: dry, pasty, thick, crumbly   → unable to determine

✱ days with menstrual bleeding   ✔ intercourse, artificial inseminations, assisted reproductive procedures

Information from physician: Ultrasound—follicle measurement (in mm) R = right ovary L = left ovary; Ovulation predictor kit: ✔ day of LH surge

Month _____ **Year** _____

Day

Cycle Day	1	2	3	4	5	6	7	8	9	10	11	12	13	14	15	16	17	18	19	20	21	22	23	24	25	26	27	28	29	30	31
cervical mucus																															
menstrual period																															
conception attempts																															
ovulation predictor kit																															
follicle size by ultrasound (mm)																															

Oral Temperature °F

Cycle Day	1	2	3	4	5	6	7	8	9	10	11	12	13	14	15	16	17	18	19	20	21	22	23	24	25	26	27	28	29	30	31
99.8																															
99.6																															
99.4																															
99.2																															
99.0																															
98.8																															
98.6																															
98.4																															
98.2																															
98.0																															
97.8																															
97.6																															
97.4																															
97.2																															
97.0																															
96.8																															

Date of ovulation _____ Transfer to the calendar section starting on page 57 for easy reference about the whole month.

Symbols:

↑ ovulatory mucus: slippery, copious, stretchy, clear   ↓ normal mucus: dry, pasty, thick, crumbly   → unable to determine

✳ days with menstrual bleeding   ✔ intercourse, artificial inseminations, assisted reproductive procedures

Information from physician: Ultrasound—follicle measurement (in mm) R = right ovary L = left ovary; Ovulation predictor kit: ✔ day of LH surge

Month _____ Year _____

Day

Cycle Day	1	2	3	4	5	6	7	8	9	10	11	12	13	14	15	16	17	18	19	20	21	22	23	24	25	26	27	28	29	30	31
cervical mucus																															
menstrual period																															
conception attempts																															
ovulation predictor kit																															
follicle size by ultrasound (mm)																															

Oral Temperature °F

Cycle Day	1	2	3	4	5	6	7	8	9	10	11	12	13	14	15	16	17	18	19	20	21	22	23	24	25	26	27	28	29	30	31
99.8																															
99.6																															
99.4																															
99.2																															
99.0																															
98.8																															
98.6																															
98.4																															
98.2																															
98.0																															
97.8																															
97.6																															
97.4																															
97.2																															
97.0																															
96.8																															

Date of ovulation _____ Transfer to the calendar section starting on page 57 for easy reference about the whole month.

Symbols:

↑ ovulatory mucus: slippery, copious, stretchy, clear ↔ normal mucus: dry, pasty, thick, crumbly → unable to determine

✻ days with menstrual bleeding ✔ intercourse, artificial inseminations, assisted reproductive procedures

Information from physician: Ultrasound—follicle measurement (in mm) R = right ovary L = left ovary; Ovulation predictor kit: ✔ day of LH surge

Month _____ Year _____

Day

Cycle Day	1	2	3	4	5	6	7	8	9	10	11	12	13	14	15	16	17	18	19	20	21	22	23	24	25	26	27	28	29	30	31
cervical mucus																															
menstrual period																															
conception attempts																															
ovulation predictor kit																															
follicle size by ultrasound (mm)																															

Oral Temperature °F

Cycle Day	1	2	3	4	5	6	7	8	9	10	11	12	13	14	15	16	17	18	19	20	21	22	23	24	25	26	27	28	29	30	31
99.8																															
99.6																															
99.4																															
99.2																															
99.0																															
98.8																															
98.6																															
98.4																															
98.2																															
98.0																															
97.8																															
97.6																															
97.4																															
97.2																															
97.0																															
96.8																															

Date of ovulation

Transfer to the calendar section starting on page 57 for easy reference about the whole month.

Symbols:

↑ ovulatory mucus: slippery, copious, stretchy, clear   ↓ normal mucus: dry, pasty, thick, crumbly   ↑ unable to determine

✱ days with menstrual bleeding   ✔ intercourse, artificial inseminations, assisted reproductive procedures

Information from physician: Ultrasound—follicle measurement (in mm) R = right ovary L = left ovary; Ovulation predictor kit: ✔ day of LH surge

Month _____ **Year** _____

Day

Cycle Day	1	2	3	4	5	6	7	8	9	10	11	12	13	14	15	16	17	18	19	20	21	22	23	24	25	26	27	28	29	30	31
cervical mucus																															
menstrual period																															
conception attempts																															
ovulation predictor kit																															
follicle size by ultrasound (mm)																															

Oral Temperature °F

Cycle Day	1	2	3	4	5	6	7	8	9	10	11	12	13	14	15	16	17	18	19	20	21	22	23	24	25	26	27	28	29	30	31
99.8																															
99.6																															
99.4																															
99.2																															
99.0																															
98.8																															
98.6																															
98.4																															
98.2																															
98.0																															
97.8																															
97.6																															
97.4																															
97.2																															
97.0																															
96.8																															

Date of ovulation _____ Transfer to the calendar section starting on page 57 for easy reference about the whole month.

Symbols:

↑ ovulatory mucus: slippery, copious, stretchy, clear ↓ normal mucus: dry, pasty, thick, crumbly → unable to determine

∗ days with menstrual bleeding ✔ intercourse, artificial inseminations, assisted reproductive procedures

Information from physician: Ultrasound—follicle measurement (in mm) R = right ovary L = left ovary; Ovulation predictor kit: ✔ day of LH surge

Month _____ Year _____

Day

Cycle Day	1	2	3	4	5	6	7	8	9	10	11	12	13	14	15	16	17	18	19	20	21	22	23	24	25	26	27	28	29	30	31
cervical mucus																															
menstrual period																															
conception attempts																															
ovulation predictor kit																															
follicle size by ultrasound (mm)																															

Oral Temperature °F

Cycle Day	1	2	3	4	5	6	7	8	9	10	11	12	13	14	15	16	17	18	19	20	21	22	23	24	25	26	27	28	29	30	31
99.8																															
99.6																															
99.4																															
99.2																															
99.0																															
98.8																															
98.6																															
98.4																															
98.2																															
98.0																															
97.8																															
97.6																															
97.4																															
97.2																															
97.0																															
96.8																															

Date of ovulation

Transfer to the calendar section starting on page 57 for easy reference about the whole month.

Symbols:

↑ ovulatory mucus: slippery, copious, stretchy, clear ↓ normal mucus: dry, pasty, thick, crumbly ↑ unable to determine

∗ days with menstrual bleeding ✔ intercourse, artificial inseminations, assisted reproductive procedures

Information from physician: Ultrasound—follicle measurement (in mm) R = right ovary L = left ovary; Ovulation predictor kit: ✔ day of LH surge

Month _____ **Year** _____

Day

Cycle Day	1	2	3	4	5	6	7	8	9	10	11	12	13	14	15	16	17	18	19	20	21	22	23	24	25	26	27	28	29	30	31
cervical mucus																															
menstrual period																															
conception attempts																															
ovulation predictor kit																															
follicle size by ultrasound (mm)																															

Oral Temperature °F

Cycle Day	1	2	3	4	5	6	7	8	9	10	11	12	13	14	15	16	17	18	19	20	21	22	23	24	25	26	27	28	29	30	31
99.8																															
99.6																															
99.4																															
99.2																															
99.0																															
98.8																															
98.6																															
98.4																															
98.2																															
98.0																															
97.8																															
97.6																															
97.4																															
97.2																															
97.0																															
96.8																															

Date of ovulation _____   Transfer to the calendar section starting on page 57 for easy reference about the whole month.

Symbols:

✚ ovulatory mucus: slippery, copious, stretchy, clear   ✦ normal mucus: dry, pasty, thick, crumbly   ✦ unable to determine

✻ days with menstrual bleeding   ✔ intercourse, artificial inseminations, assisted reproductive procedures

Information from physician: Ultrasound—follicle measurement (in mm) R = right ovary L = left ovary; Ovulation predictor kit: ✔ day of LH surge

Month_____ **Year**___

Day

Cycle Day	1	2	3	4	5	6	7	8	9	10	11	12	13	14	15	16	17	18	19	20	21	22	23	24	25	26	27	28	29	30	31
cervical mucus																															
menstrual period																															
conception attempts																															
ovulation predictor kit																															
follicle size by ultrasound (mm)																															

Oral Temperature °F

Cycle Day	1	2	3	4	5	6	7	8	9	10	11	12	13	14	15	16	17	18	19	20	21	22	23	24	25	26	27	28	29	30	31
99.8																															
99.6																															
99.4																															
99.2																															
99.0																															
98.8																															
98.6																															
98.4																															
98.2																															
98.0																															
97.8																															
97.6																															
97.4																															
97.2																															
97.0																															
96.8																															

Date of ovulation _____ Transfer to the calendar section starting on page 57 for easy reference about the whole month.

Symbols:

↑ ovulatory mucus: slippery, copious, stretchy, clear   ↓ normal mucus: dry, pasty, thick, crumbly   → unable to determine

✳ days with menstrual bleeding   ✔ intercourse, artificial inseminations, assisted reproductive procedures

Information from physician: Ultrasound—follicle measurement (in mm) R = right ovary L = left ovary; Ovulation predictor kit: ✔ day of LH surge

Month_____ Year_____

Day

Cycle Day	1	2	3	4	5	6	7	8	9	10	11	12	13	14	15	16	17	18	19	20	21	22	23	24	25	26	27	28	29	30	31
cervical mucus																															
menstrual period																															
conception attempts																															
ovulation predictor kit																															
follicle size by ultrasound (mm)																															

Oral Temperature °F

Cycle Day	1	2	3	4	5	6	7	8	9	10	11	12	13	14	15	16	17	18	19	20	21	22	23	24	25	26	27	28	29	30	31
99.8																															
99.6																															
99.4																															
99.2																															
99.0																															
98.8																															
98.6																															
98.4																															
98.2																															
98.0																															
97.8																															
97.6																															
97.4																															
97.2																															
97.0																															
96.8																															

Date of ovulation _____

Transfer to the calendar section starting on page 57 for easy reference about the whole month.

Symbols:

↑ ovulatory mucus: slippery, copious, stretchy, clear   ↓ normal mucus: dry, pasty, thick, crumbly   ↦ unable to determine

＊ days with menstrual bleeding   ✔ intercourse, artificial inseminations, assisted reproductive procedures

Information from physician: Ultrasound—follicle measurement (in mm) R = right ovary L = left ovary; Ovulation predictor kit: ✔ day of LH surge

Month _____   Year _____

Day

Cycle Day	1	2	3	4	5	6	7	8	9	10	11	12	13	14	15	16	17	18	19	20	21	22	23	24	25	26	27	28	29	30	31
cervical mucus																															
menstrual period																															
conception attempts																															
ovulation predictor kit																															
follicle size by ultrasound (mm)																															

Oral Temperature °F

Cycle Day	1	2	3	4	5	6	7	8	9	10	11	12	13	14	15	16	17	18	19	20	21	22	23	24	25	26	27	28	29	30	31
99.8																															
99.6																															
99.4																															
99.2																															
99.0																															
98.8																															
98.6																															
98.4																															
98.2																															
98.0																															
97.8																															
97.6																															
97.4																															
97.2																															
97.0																															
96.8																															

Date of ovulation _____   Transfer to the calendar section starting on page 57 for easy reference about the whole month.

Symbols:

↑ ovulatory mucus: slippery, copious, stretchy, clear   ↓ normal mucus: dry, pasty, thick, crumbly   → unable to determine

✻ days with menstrual bleeding   ✔ intercourse, artificial inseminations, assisted reproductive procedures

Information from physician: Ultrasound—follicle measurement (in mm) R = right ovary L = left ovary; Ovulation predictor kit: ✔ day of LH surge

Month_____ Year____

Day

Cycle Day	1	2	3	4	5	6	7	8	9	10	11	12	13	14	15	16	17	18	19	20	21	22	23	24	25	26	27	28	29	30	31
cervical mucus																															
menstrual period																															
conception attempts																															
ovulation predictor kit																															
follicle size by ultrasound (mm)																															

Oral Temperature °F

Cycle Day	1	2	3	4	5	6	7	8	9	10	11	12	13	14	15	16	17	18	19	20	21	22	23	24	25	26	27	28	29	30	31
99.8																															
99.6																															
99.4																															
99.2																															
99.0																															
98.8																															
98.6																															
98.4																															
98.2																															
98.0																															
97.8																															
97.6																															
97.4																															
97.2																															
97.0																															
96.8																															

Date of ovulation

Transfer to the calendar section starting on page 57 for easy reference about the whole month.

Symbols:

↑ ovulatory mucus: slippery, copious, stretchy, clear ↓ normal mucus: dry, pasty, thick, crumbly → unable to determine

* days with menstrual bleeding ✔ intercourse, artificial inseminations, assisted reproductive procedures

Information from physician: Ultrasound—follicle measurement (in mm) R = right ovary L = left ovary; Ovulation predictor kit: ✔ day of LH surge

Month _____ Year _____

Day

Cycle Day	1	2	3	4	5	6	7	8	9	10	11	12	13	14	15	16	17	18	19	20	21	22	23	24	25	26	27	28	29	30	31
cervical mucus																															
menstrual period																															
conception attempts																															
ovulation predictor kit																															
follicle size by ultrasound (mm)																															

Oral Temperature °F

Cycle Day	1	2	3	4	5	6	7	8	9	10	11	12	13	14	15	16	17	18	19	20	21	22	23	24	25	26	27	28	29	30	31
99.8																															
99.6																															
99.4																															
99.2																															
99.0																															
98.8																															
98.6																															
98.4																															
98.2																															
98.0																															
97.8																															
97.6																															
97.4																															
97.2																															
97.0																															
96.8																															

Date of ovulation

Transfer to the calendar section starting on page 57 for easy reference about the whole month.

Symbols:

↑ ovulatory mucus: slippery, copious, stretchy, clear   ↓ normal mucus: dry, pasty, thick, crumbly   ↛ unable to determine

✳ days with menstrual bleeding   ✔ intercourse, artificial inseminations, assisted reproductive procedures

Information from physician: Ultrasound—follicle measurement (in mm)   R = right ovary   L = left ovary; Ovulation predictor kit: ✔ day of LH surge

Month_____ Year____

Day

Cycle Day	1	2	3	4	5	6	7	8	9	10	11	12	13	14	15	16	17	18	19	20	21	22	23	24	25	26	27	28	29	30	31
cervical mucus																															
menstrual period																															
conception attempts																															
ovulation predictor kit																															
follicle size by ultrasound (mm)																															

Oral Temperature °F

Cycle Day	1	2	3	4	5	6	7	8	9	10	11	12	13	14	15	16	17	18	19	20	21	22	23	24	25	26	27	28	29	30	31
99.8																															
99.6																															
99.4																															
99.2																															
99.0																															
98.8																															
98.6																															
98.4																															
98.2																															
98.0																															
97.8																															
97.6																															
97.4																															
97.2																															
97.0																															
96.8																															

Date of ovulation_____

Transfer to the calendar section starting on page 57 for easy reference about the whole month.

Symbols:

↑ ovulatory mucus: slippery, copious, stretchy, clear   ↓ normal mucus: dry, pasty, thick, crumbly   → unable to determine

✳ days with menstrual bleeding   ✔ intercourse, artificial inseminations, assisted reproductive procedures

Information from physician: Ultrasound—follicle measurement (in mm) R = right ovary L = left ovary; Ovulation predictor kit: ✔ day of LH surge

Month _____ Year _____

Day

Cycle Day	1	2	3	4	5	6	7	8	9	10	11	12	13	14	15	16	17	18	19	20	21	22	23	24	25	26	27	28	29	30	31
cervical mucus																															
menstrual period																															
conception attempts																															
ovulation predictor kit																															
follicle size by ultrasound (mm)																															

Oral Temperature °F

Cycle Day	1	2	3	4	5	6	7	8	9	10	11	12	13	14	15	16	17	18	19	20	21	22	23	24	25	26	27	28	29	30	31
99.8																															
99.6																															
99.4																															
99.2																															
99.0																															
98.8																															
98.6																															
98.4																															
98.2																															
98.0																															
97.8																															
97.6																															
97.4																															
97.2																															
97.0																															
96.8																															

Date of ovulation _____ Transfer to the calendar section starting on page 57 for easy reference about the whole month.

Symbols:

↑ ovulatory mucus: slippery, copious, stretchy, clear ↓ normal mucus: dry, pasty, thick, crumbly → unable to determine

* days with menstrual bleeding ✔ intercourse, artificial inseminations, assisted reproductive procedures

Information from physician: Ultrasound—follicle measurement (in mm) R = right ovary L = left ovary; Ovulation predictor kit: ✔ day of LH surge

Month _____ **Year** _____

Day

Cycle Day	1	2	3	4	5	6	7	8	9	10	11	12	13	14	15	16	17	18	19	20	21	22	23	24	25	26	27	28	29	30	31
cervical mucus																															
menstrual period																															
conception attempts																															
ovulation predictor kit																															
follicle size by ultrasound (mm)																															

Oral Temperature °F

Cycle Day	1	2	3	4	5	6	7	8	9	10	11	12	13	14	15	16	17	18	19	20	21	22	23	24	25	26	27	28	29	30	31
99.8																															
99.6																															
99.4																															
99.2																															
99.0																															
98.8																															
98.6																															
98.4																															
98.2																															
98.0																															
97.8																															
97.6																															
97.4																															
97.2																															
97.0																															
96.8																															

Date of ovulation _____ Transfer to the calendar section starting on page 57 for easy reference about the whole month.

Symbols:

↑ ovulatory mucus: slippery, copious, stretchy, clear   ↓ normal mucus: dry, pasty, thick, crumbly   → unable to determine

* days with menstrual bleeding   ✔ intercourse, artificial inseminations, assisted reproductive procedures

Information from physician: Ultrasound—follicle measurement (in mm) R = right ovary L = left ovary; Ovulation predictor kit: ✔ day of LH surge

Month _____ Year _____

Day

Cycle Day	1	2	3	4	5	6	7	8	9	10	11	12	13	14	15	16	17	18	19	20	21	22	23	24	25	26	27	28	29	30	31
cervical mucus																															
menstrual period																															
conception attempts																															
ovulation predictor kit																															
follicle size by ultrasound (mm)																															

Oral Temperature °F

Cycle Day	1	2	3	4	5	6	7	8	9	10	11	12	13	14	15	16	17	18	19	20	21	22	23	24	25	26	27	28	29	30	31
99.8																															
99.6																															
99.4																															
99.2																															
99.0																															
98.8																															
98.6																															
98.4																															
98.2																															
98.0																															
97.8																															
97.6																															
97.4																															
97.2																															
97.0																															
96.8																															

Date of ovulation

Transfer to the calendar section starting on page 57 for easy reference about the whole month.

Symbols:

↑ ovulatory mucus: slippery, copious, stretchy, clear ↓ normal mucus: dry, pasty, thick, crumbly → unable to determine

✳ days with menstrual bleeding ✔ intercourse, artificial inseminations, assisted reproductive procedures

Information from physician: Ultrasound—follicle measurement (in mm) R = right ovary L = left ovary; Ovulation predictor kit: ✔ day of LH surge

Month _____ **Year** _____

Day

Cycle Day

	1	2	3	4	5	6	7	8	9	10	11	12	13	14	15	16	17	18	19	20	21	22	23	24	25	26	27	28	29	30	31
cervical mucus																															
menstrual period																															
conception attempts																															
ovulation predictor kit																															
follicle size by ultrasound (mm)																															

Oral Temperature °F

Cycle Day

	1	2	3	4	5	6	7	8	9	10	11	12	13	14	15	16	17	18	19	20	21	22	23	24	25	26	27	28	29	30	31
99.8																															
99.6																															
99.4																															
99.2																															
99.0																															
98.8																															
98.6																															
98.4																															
98.2																															
98.0																															
97.8																															
97.6																															
97.4																															
97.2																															
97.0																															
96.8																															

Date of ovulation

Transfer to the calendar section starting on page 57 for easy reference about the whole month.

Symbols:

↑ ovulatory mucus: slippery, copious, stretchy, clear   ↓ normal mucus: dry, pasty, thick, crumbly   → unable to determine

✴ days with menstrual bleeding   ✔ intercourse, artificial inseminations, assisted reproductive procedures

Information from physician: Ultrasound—follicle measurement (in mm) R = right ovary L = left ovary; Ovulation predictor kit: ✔ day of LH surge

Month_____ Year_____

Day

Cycle Day	1	2	3	4	5	6	7	8	9	10	11	12	13	14	15	16	17	18	19	20	21	22	23	24	25	26	27	28	29	30	31
cervical mucus																															
menstrual period																															
conception attempts																															
ovulation predictor kit																															
follicle size by ultrasound (mm)																															

Oral Temperature °F

Cycle Day	1	2	3	4	5	6	7	8	9	10	11	12	13	14	15	16	17	18	19	20	21	22	23	24	25	26	27	28	29	30	31
99.8																															
99.6																															
99.4																															
99.2																															
99.0																															
98.8																															
98.6																															
98.4																															
98.2																															
98.0																															
97.8																															
97.6																															
97.4																															
97.2																															
97.0																															
96.8																															

Date of ovulation _____ Transfer to the calendar section starting on page 57 for easy reference about the whole month.

Symbols:

↑ ovulatory mucus: slippery, copious, stretchy, clear ↓ normal mucus: dry, pasty, thick, crumbly → unable to determine

✻ days with menstrual bleeding ✔ intercourse, artificial inseminations, assisted reproductive procedures

Information from physician: Ultrasound—follicle measurement (in mm) R = right ovary L = left ovary; Ovulation predictor kit: ✔ day of LH surge

Month _____ **Year** _____

Day

Cycle Day	1	2	3	4	5	6	7	8	9	10	11	12	13	14	15	16	17	18	19	20	21	22	23	24	25	26	27	28	29	30	31
cervical mucus																															
menstrual period																															
conception attempts																															
ovulation predictor kit																															
follicle size by ultrasound (mm)																															

Oral Temperature °F

Cycle Day	1	2	3	4	5	6	7	8	9	10	11	12	13	14	15	16	17	18	19	20	21	22	23	24	25	26	27	28	29	30	31
99.8																															
99.6																															
99.4																															
99.2																															
99.0																															
98.8																															
98.6																															
98.4																															
98.2																															
98.0																															
97.8																															
97.6																															
97.4																															
97.2																															
97.0																															
96.8																															

Date of ovulation _____

Transfer to the calendar section starting on page 57 for easy reference about the whole month.

Symbols:

↑ ovulatory mucus: slippery, copious, stretchy, clear   ↓ normal mucus: dry, pasty, thick, crumbly   → unable to determine

✱ days with menstrual bleeding   ✔ intercourse, artificial inseminations, assisted reproductive procedures

Information from physician: Ultrasound—follicle measurement (in mm) R = right ovary L = left ovary; Ovulation predictor kit: ✔ day of LH surge

Month _____ Year _____

Day

Cycle Day	1 2 3 4 5 6 7 8 9 10 11 12 13 14 15 16 17 18 19 20 21 22 23 24 25 26 27 28 29 30 31
cervical mucus	
menstrual period	
conception attempts	
ovulation predictor kit	
follicle size by ultrasound (mm)	

Oral Temperature °F

Cycle Day	1 2 3 4 5 6 7 8 9 10 11 12 13 14 15 16 17 18 19 20 21 22 23 24 25 26 27 28 29 30 31
99.8	
99.6	
99.4	
99.2	
99.0	
98.8	
98.6	
98.4	
98.2	
98.0	
97.8	
97.6	
97.4	
97.2	
97.0	
96.8	

Date of ovulation _____

Transfer to the calendar section starting on page 57 for easy reference about the whole month.

Symbols:

↑ ovulatory mucus: slippery, copious, stretchy, clear → normal mucus: dry, pasty, thick, crumbly ↛ unable to determine

✷ days with menstrual bleeding ✔ intercourse, artificial inseminations, assisted reproductive procedures

Information from physician: Ultrasound—follicle measurement (in mm) R = right ovary L = left ovary; Ovulation predictor kit: ✔ day of LH surge

Month _____ Year _____

Day

Cycle Day	1	2	3	4	5	6	7	8	9	10	11	12	13	14	15	16	17	18	19	20	21	22	23	24	25	26	27	28	29	30	31
cervical mucus																															
menstrual period																															
conception attempts																															
ovulation predictor kit																															
follicle size by ultrasound (mm)																															

Oral Temperature °F

Cycle Day	1	2	3	4	5	6	7	8	9	10	11	12	13	14	15	16	17	18	19	20	21	22	23	24	25	26	27	28	29	30	31
99.8																															
99.6																															
99.4																															
99.2																															
99.0																															
98.8																															
98.6																															
98.4																															
98.2																															
98.0																															
97.8																															
97.6																															
97.4																															
97.2																															
97.0																															
96.8																															

Date of ovulation _____ Transfer to the calendar section starting on page 57 for easy reference about the whole month.

Symbols:

↑ ovulatory mucus: slippery, copious, stretchy, clear   ↓ normal mucus: dry, pasty, thick, crumbly   → unable to determine

✳ days with menstrual bleeding   ✔ intercourse, artificial inseminations, assisted reproductive procedures

Information from physician: Ultrasound —follicle measurement (in mm) R = right ovary L = left ovary; Ovulation predictor kit: ✔ day of LH surge

Month _____ Year _____

Day

Cycle Day	1	2	3	4	5	6	7	8	9	10	11	12	13	14	15	16	17	18	19	20	21	22	23	24	25	26	27	28	29	30	31
cervical mucus																															
menstrual period																															
conception attempts																															
ovulation predictor kit																															
follicle size by ultrasound (mm)																															

Oral Temperature °F

Cycle Day	1	2	3	4	5	6	7	8	9	10	11	12	13	14	15	16	17	18	19	20	21	22	23	24	25	26	27	28	29	30	31
99.8																															
99.6																															
99.4																															
99.2																															
99.0																															
98.8																															
98.6																															
98.4																															
98.2																															
98.0																															
97.8																															
97.6																															
97.4																															
97.2																															
97.0																															
96.8																															

Date of ovulation _____

Transfer to the calendar section starting on page 57 for easy reference about the whole month.

Symbols:

↑ ovulatory mucus: slippery, copious, stretchy, clear   ↓ normal mucus: dry, pasty, thick, crumbly   → unable to determine

✳ days with menstrual bleeding   ✔ intercourse, artificial inseminations, assisted reproductive procedures

Information from physician: Ultrasound—follicle measurement (in mm) R = right ovary L = left ovary; Ovulation predictor kit: ✔ day of LH surge

The Calendar

Once you have charted a whole cycle on Your Detailed Monthly Charts, transfer major events onto this calendar. This might include dates of inseminations, procedures, ovulation, medicines, or appointments. The resulting calendar will reveal all of your key events for that month at a glance. Why not just use Your Detailed Monthly Charts themselves? That's fine, too—if it's easier for you. However, once you've charted every detail of a given cycle—for instance, temperatures, cervical mucus scoring, hormone levels, and more—and you know when you ovulated, it's nice to abstract that information onto the calendar. Then, the date the main events occurred will be readily visible. This can be useful to figure out when you might want to get a pregnancy test, or other diagnostic procedures.

Month

Year

Sunday	Monday	Tuesday	Wednesday	Thursday	Friday	Saturday

Month

Year

Sunday	Monday	Tuesday	Wednesday	Thursday	Friday	Saturday

Month

Year

Sunday	Monday	Tuesday	Wednesday	Thursday	Friday	Saturday

Month

Year

Sunday	Monday	Tuesday	Wednesday	Thursday	Friday	Saturday

Month

Year

Sunday	Monday	Tuesday	Wednesday	Thursday	Friday	Saturday

Month

Year

Sunday	Monday	Tuesday	Wednesday	Thursday	Friday	Saturday

Month

Year

Sunday	Monday	Tuesday	Wednesday	Thursday	Friday	Saturday

Month

Year

Sunday	Monday	Tuesday	Wednesday	Thursday	Friday	Saturday

Month

Year

Sunday	Monday	Tuesday	Wednesday	Thursday	Friday	Saturday

Month

Year

Sunday	Monday	Tuesday	Wednesday	Thursday	Friday	Saturday

Month

Year

Sunday	Monday	Tuesday	Wednesday	Thursday	Friday	Saturday

Month

Year

Sunday	Monday	Tuesday	Wednesday	Thursday	Friday	Saturday

Month

Year

Sunday	Monday	Tuesday	Wednesday	Thursday	Friday	Saturday

Month

Year

Sunday	Monday	Tuesday	Wednesday	Thursday	Friday	Saturday

Month

Year

Sunday	Monday	Tuesday	Wednesday	Thursday	Friday	Saturday

Month

Year

Sunday	Monday	Tuesday	Wednesday	Thursday	Friday	Saturday

Month

Year

Sunday	Monday	Tuesday	Wednesday	Thursday	Friday	Saturday

Month

Year

Sunday	Monday	Tuesday	Wednesday	Thursday	Friday	Saturday

Month

Year

Sunday	Monday	Tuesday	Wednesday	Thursday	Friday	Saturday

Month

Year

Sunday	Monday	Tuesday	Wednesday	Thursday	Friday	Saturday

Month   **Year**

	Sunday	Monday	Tuesday	Wednesday	Thursday	Friday	Saturday

Month

Year

Sunday	Monday	Tuesday	Wednesday	Thursday	Friday	Saturday

Month

Year

Sunday	Monday	Tuesday	Wednesday	Thursday	Friday	Saturday

Month

Year

Sunday	Monday	Tuesday	Wednesday	Thursday	Friday	Saturday

Infertility Treatment

There is a veritable smorgasbord of treatment available for obstacles to both male and female infertility. We've already discussed the array of methods available to diagnose fertility problems, and there is an even larger array of medications, procedures, surgeries, combination regimens, and more to treat them. Each person undergoing infertility treatment will likely have a unique assortment of treatments: some may have one simple, low-tech treatment while others may have a variety of complex high-tech treatments. In view of this diversity, the organizer is set up to allow you maximal flexibility in recording your treatments; there are multiple charts on which you can record your customized treatment regimen. If your infertility treatment includes medications, chart them on the Infertility Medications chart; if you undergo procedures or ARTs, chart them on the Infertility Procedures chart. Knowing which steps you've taken to overcome your obstacles to fertility and when you've taken them will keep you organized and serve as a great reference along your path to parenthood.

Infertility Medications

This section houses tables for information about your infertility medications. You may not take any medications or you may take all of them: use this table to suit your specific treatment regimen. For each cycle, write down what medicines you are supposed to take on each cycle day, the dose and the route, and then check each off as you take it. (A handy way to be sure you do not miss a dose! Compliance with infertility treatment regimens is crucial.) The charts are flexible enough to include medications for ovulation induction or any other therapies. In some treatment regimens, blood hormone levels are measured frequently to determine the proper doses. There is room on these charts for you to note your hormone levels, if you choose (you can also note them on Your Detailed Monthly Charts).

Note in the comments column how you feel, special instructions your physician has given you, or if you have side effects that should be brought to the attention of your physician.

SOME COMMON INFERTILITY MEDICATIONS

Function of Medication	Generic Name
Reduction of prolactin level	bromocriptine mesylate (Parlodel)
Turns off release of GnRH to prevent premature LH surge; GnRH agonist	leuprolide acetate (Lupron), nafarelin acetate (Synarel), buserelin
Induces ovulation	clomiphene citrate (Clomid, Serophene)
Inhibits pituitary production of FSH and LH to treat endometriosis	danocrine (Danazol)
Induces ovulation; FSH extract	FSH (Metrodin)
Induces ovulation; recombinant form of FSH	urofollitropin (Fertinex)
Turns off release of GnRH to prevent premature LH surge. May be used in patients with amenorrhea also; GnRH	GnRH (Lutrepulse)
Induces ovulation of prepared eggs by simulating LH surge; sometimes used in males to stimulate testosterone production	human chorionic gonadotropin (hCG) (Pregnyl, Profasi)

Function of Medication	Generic Name
Induces ovulation; this drug is combination LH and FSH extract	Human menopausal gonadotropins (HMG) (Pergonal, Humegon, Repronex)
Natural progesterone used as supplement in cases of luteal phase insufficiency, and after ARTs	progesterone (Crinone), hydroxyprogesterone caproate
Synthetic progesterones used as contraceptives, to regulate cycle prior to ARTs, treatment for menstrual irregularity, and to diagnose hormone problems (with progesterone withdrawal test	medroxyprogesterone acetate (Provera), norethidrone acetate (Norlutate), oral contraceptives

Infertility Medications

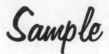

Cycle Day Number/ Date	Medication	Dose/Route	Taken?	Comments	Hormone Test Results
1.					
2.					
3. 3/4/99	clomiphene citrate	50mg/by mouth	✔		n/a
4. 3/5/99	clomiphene citrate	50mg/by mouth	✔	felt nauseated	n/a
5. 3/6/99	clomiphene citrate	50mg/by mouth	✔	better today	n/a
6. 3/7/99	clomiphene citrate	50mg/by mouth	✔		n/a
7. 3/8/99	clomiphene citrate	50mg/by mouth	✔		n/a
8.					
9.					
10.					
11.					
12.	start daily LH urine testing per Dr. Jones				
13.					
14.					
15.					
16.					
17.					
18.					
19.					
20.					
21.					
22.					
23.					
24.					
25.					
26.					
27.					
28.					

Infertility Medications

Cycle Day Number/ Date	Medication	Dose/Route	Taken?	Comments	Hormone Test Results
1.					
2.					
3.					
4.					
5.					
6.					
7.					
8.					
9.					
10.					
11.					
12.					
13.					
14.					
15.					
16.					
17.					
18.					
19.					
20.					
21.					
22.					
23.					
24.					
25.					
26.					
27.					
28.					

Infertility Medications

Cycle Day Number/ Date	Medication	Dose/Route	Taken?	Comments	Hormone Test Results
1.					
2.					
3.					
4.					
5.					
6.					
7.					
8.					
9.					
10.					
11.					
12.					
13.					
14.					
15.					
16.					
17.					
18.					
19.					
20.					
21.					
22.					
23.					
24.					
25.					
26.					
27.					
28.					

Infertility Medications

Cycle Day Number/ Date	Medication	Dose/Route	Taken?	Comments	Hormone Test Results
1.					
2.					
3.					
4.					
5.					
6.					
7.					
8.					
9.					
10.					
11.					
12.					
13.					
14.					
15.					
16.					
17.					
18.					
19.					
20.					
21.					
22.					
23.					
24.					
25.					
26.					
27.					
28.					

Infertility Medications

Cycle Day Number/ Date	Medication	Dose/Route	Taken?	Comments	Hormone Test Results
1.					
2.					
3.					
4.					
5.					
6.					
7.					
8.					
9.					
10.					
11.					
12.					
13.					
14.					
15.					
16.					
17.					
18.					
19.					
20.					
21.					
22.					
23.					
24.					
25.					
26.					
27.					
28.					

Infertility Medications

Cycle Day Number/ Date	Medication	Dose/Route	Taken?	Comments	Hormone Test Results
1.					
2.					
3.					
4.					
5.					
6.					
7.					
8.					
9.					
10.					
11.					
12.					
13.					
14.					
15.					
16.					
17.					
18.					
19.					
20.					
21.					
22.					
23.					
24.					
25.					
26.					
27.					
28.					

Infertility Medications

Cycle Day Number/ Date	Medication	Dose/Route	Taken?	Comments	Hormone Test Results
1.					
2.					
3.					
4.					
5.					
6.					
7.					
8.					
9.					
10.					
11.					
12.					
13.					
14.					
15.					
16.					
17.					
18.					
19.					
20.					
21.					
22.					
23.					
24.					
25.					
26.					
27.					
28.					

Infertility Procedures

Many infertility procedures are available to assist you in becoming pregnant; you, your partner, and your physician will decide which ones are right for you. Some of the procedures available right now are artificial insemination (AI), intrauterine insemination (IUI), in vitro fertilization (IVF), gamete intrafallopian transfer (GIFT), and zygote intrafallopian transfer (ZIFT). The glossary introduces these to you; other books and your physician can give you a more detailed understanding of the advantages and disadvantages of each in your special case. If you undertake any of these procedures, you can chart the details here. This will help you remember what you have done and will give you a sense of accomplishment along your fertility journey. Like the preceding treatment section, this chart is designed to be compatible with any assortment of procedures you might have.

HOW MANY PEOPLE ARE SUBFERTILE?

The National Center for Health Statistics indicates that in 1995 there were 6.1 million women ages 15 to 44 in the United States with impaired ability to have children. They report that in the United States, 9 million women used infertility services. The World Health Organization indicates that globally approximately 50 to 80 million couples have some difficulty with their fertility. So while we may often feel isolated in our difficulty to bear a child, we are in quite good company statistically speaking.

It is important to remember, though, that most people will get pregnant over time. If you took a group of 100 perfectly fertile women in their early 20s, with perfectly fertile partners, the first month they tried to conceive, about 20 percent of them (20) would get pregnant. The next month, about 20 percent of the remaining 80 would become pregnant (16). And so on. Each cycle, there is a pretty stable and constant 20 percent rate of conception. About 85 percent of perfectly fertile women trying to conceive would become pregnant within the first year, and about 15 percent would not. Within two years about 95 percent of them would be pregnant. And they are perfectly fertile! Not everyone gets pregnant at first, but over time, most will. As we age, this per cycle conception rate decreases some, but the principle remains the same. So even if you do not become pregnant right away, you and your partner may be completely normal, with no fertility problem whatsoever. Depending on your circumstances, your physician may even recommend that you hold off on infertility treatments for some time, and keep trying naturally.

Infertility Treatments

Sample

Date	Procedure		If applicable, Number of Eggs Aspirated/Embryos Implanted/Location Implanted	Comments
3/10/99	❏ AI	☑ IUI	*not applicable*	*Went well! Slightly uncomfortable*
	❏ GIFT	❏ ZIFT		*when catheter inserted, but otherwise*
	❏ IVF	❏ other		*OK. Dr Jones said there was no*
				bleeding, which is a good sign!
	❏ AI	❏ IUI		
	❏ GIFT	❏ ZIFT		
	❏ IVF	❏ other		
	❏ AI	❏ IUI		
	❏ GIFT	❏ ZIFT		
	❏ IVF	❏ other		
	❏ AI	❏ IUI		
	❏ GIFT	❏ ZIFT		
	❏ IVF	❏ other		
	❏ AI	❏ IUI		
	❏ GIFT	❏ ZIFT		
	❏ IVF	❏ other		
	❏ AI	❏ IUI		
	❏ GIFT	❏ ZIFT		
	❏ IVF	❏ other		

AI = artificial insemination; IUI = intrauterine insemination; GIFT = gamete intrafollopian transfer; ZIFT = zygote intrafallopian transfer; IVF = in vitro fertilization

Infertility Treatments

Date	Procedure		If applicable, Number of Eggs Aspirated/Embryos Implanted/Location Implanted	Comments
_____	❏ AI	❏ IUI	_____	_____
_____	❏ GIFT	❏ ZIFT	_____	_____
_____	❏ IVF	❏ other	_____	_____
_____	❏ AI	❏ IUI	_____	_____
_____	❏ GIFT	❏ ZIFT	_____	_____
_____	❏ IVF	❏ other	_____	_____
_____	❏ AI	❏ IUI	_____	_____
_____	❏ GIFT	❏ ZIFT	_____	_____
_____	❏ IVF	❏ other	_____	_____
_____	❏ AI	❏ IUI	_____	_____
_____	❏ GIFT	❏ ZIFT	_____	_____
_____	❏ IVF	❏ other	_____	_____
_____	❏ AI	❏ IUI	_____	_____
_____	❏ GIFT	❏ ZIFT	_____	_____
_____	❏ IVF	❏ other	_____	_____
_____	❏ AI	❏ IUI	_____	_____
_____	❏ GIFT	❏ ZIFT	_____	_____
_____	❏ IVF	❏ other	_____	_____

AI = artificial insemination; IUI = intrauterine insemination; GIFT = gamete intrafollopian transfer; ZIFT = zygote intrafallopian transfer; IVF = in vitro fertilization

Infertility Treatments

Date	Procedure		If applicable, Number of Eggs Aspirated/Embryos Implanted/Location Implanted	Comments
_____	❏ AI	❏ IUI		
_____	❏ GIFT	❏ ZIFT		
_____	❏ IVF	❏ other		
_____	❏ AI	❏ IUI		
_____	❏ GIFT	❏ ZIFT		
_____	❏ IVF	❏ other		
_____	❏ AI	❏ IUI		
_____	❏ GIFT	❏ ZIFT		
_____	❏ IVF	❏ other		
_____	❏ AI	❏ IUI		
_____	❏ GIFT	❏ ZIFT		
_____	❏ IVF	❏ other		
_____	❏ AI	❏ IUI		
_____	❏ GIFT	❏ ZIFT		
_____	❏ IVF	❏ other		
_____	❏ AI	❏ IUI		
_____	❏ GIFT	❏ ZIFT		
_____	❏ IVF	❏ other		

AI = artificial insemination; IUI = intrauterine insemination; GIFT = gamete intrafollopian transfer; ZIFT = zygote intrafallopian transfer; IVF = in vitro fertilization

Infertility Treatments

Date	Procedure		If applicable, Number of Eggs Aspirated/Embryos Implanted/Location Implanted	Comments
_____	❑ AI	❑ IUI	_____	_____
_____	❑ GIFT	❑ ZIFT	_____	_____
_____	❑ IVF	❑ other	_____	_____
_____	❑ AI	❑ IUI	_____	_____
_____	❑ GIFT	❑ ZIFT	_____	_____
_____	❑ IVF	❑ other	_____	_____
_____	❑ AI	❑ IUI	_____	_____
_____	❑ GIFT	❑ ZIFT	_____	_____
_____	❑ IVF	❑ other	_____	_____
_____	❑ AI	❑ IUI	_____	_____
_____	❑ GIFT	❑ ZIFT	_____	_____
_____	❑ IVF	❑ other	_____	_____
_____	❑ AI	❑ IUI	_____	_____
_____	❑ GIFT	❑ ZIFT	_____	_____
_____	❑ IVF	❑ other	_____	_____
_____	❑ AI	❑ IUI	_____	_____
_____	❑ GIFT	❑ ZIFT	_____	_____
_____	❑ IVF	❑ other	_____	_____

AI = artificial insemination; IUI = intrauterine insemination; GIFT = gamete intrafollopian transfer; ZIFT = zygote intrafallopian transfer; IVF = in vitro fertilization

Infertility Treatments

Date	Procedure		If applicable, Number of Eggs Aspirated/Embryos Implanted/Location Implanted	Comments
	❑ AI	❑ IUI		
	❑ GIFT	❑ ZIFT		
	❑ IVF	❑ other		
	❑ AI	❑ IUI		
	❑ GIFT	❑ ZIFT		
	❑ IVF	❑ other		
	❑ AI	❑ IUI		
	❑ GIFT	❑ ZIFT		
	❑ IVF	❑ other		
	❑ AI	❑ IUI		
	❑ GIFT	❑ ZIFT		
	❑ IVF	❑ other		
	❑ AI	❑ IUI		
	❑ GIFT	❑ ZIFT		
	❑ IVF	❑ other		
	❑ AI	❑ IUI		
	❑ GIFT	❑ ZIFT		
	❑ IVF	❑ other		

AI = artificial insemination; IUI = intrauterine insemination; GIFT = gamete intrafollopian transfer; ZIFT = zygote intrafallopian transfer; IVF = in vitro fertilization

Infertility Treatments

Date	Procedure		If applicable, Number of Eggs Aspirated/Embryos Implanted/Location Implanted	Comments
_____	❑ AI	❑ IUI	_____	_____
_____	❑ GIFT	❑ ZIFT	_____	_____
_____	❑ IVF	❑ other	_____	_____
_____			_____	_____
_____	❑ AI	❑ IUI	_____	_____
_____	❑ GIFT	❑ ZIFT	_____	_____
_____	❑ IVF	❑ other	_____	_____
_____			_____	_____
_____	❑ AI	❑ IUI	_____	_____
_____	❑ GIFT	❑ ZIFT	_____	_____
_____	❑ IVF	❑ other	_____	_____
_____			_____	_____
_____	❑ AI	❑ IUI	_____	_____
_____	❑ GIFT	❑ ZIFT	_____	_____
_____	❑ IVF	❑ other	_____	_____
_____			_____	_____
_____	❑ AI	❑ IUI	_____	_____
_____	❑ GIFT	❑ ZIFT	_____	_____
_____	❑ IVF	❑ other	_____	_____
_____			_____	_____
_____	❑ AI	❑ IUI	_____	_____
_____	❑ GIFT	❑ ZIFT	_____	_____
_____	❑ IVF	❑ other	_____	_____
_____			_____	_____

AI = artificial insemination; IUI = intrauterine insemination; GIFT = gamete intrafollopian transfer; ZIFT = zygote intrafallopian transfer; IVF = in vitro fertilization

Infertility Treatments

Date	Procedure		If applicable, Number of Eggs Aspirated/Embryos Implanted/Location Implanted	Comments
_____	❏ AI	❏ IUI	_____	_____
_____	❏ GIFT	❏ ZIFT	_____	
_____	❏ IVF	❏ other	_____	_____
_____			_____	_____
_____	❏ AI	❏ IUI	_____	_____
_____	❏ GIFT	❏ ZIFT	_____	
_____	❏ IVF	❏ other	_____	_____
_____			_____	_____
_____	❏ AI	❏ IUI	_____	_____
_____	❏ GIFT	❏ ZIFT	_____	
_____	❏ IVF	❏ other	_____	_____
_____			_____	_____
_____	❏ AI	❏ IUI	_____	_____
_____	❏ GIFT	❏ ZIFT	_____	
_____	❏ IVF	❏ other	_____	_____
_____			_____	_____
_____	❏ AI	❏ IUI	_____	_____
_____	❏ GIFT	❏ ZIFT	_____	
_____	❏ IVF	❏ other	_____	_____
_____			_____	_____
_____	❏ AI	❏ IUI	_____	_____
_____	❏ GIFT	❏ ZIFT	_____	
_____	❏ IVF	❏ other	_____	_____
_____			_____	_____

AI = artificial insemination; IUI = intrauterine insemination; GIFT = gamete intrafollopian transfer; ZIFT = zygote intrafallopian transfer; IVF = in vitro fertilization

Infertility Treatments

Date	Procedure		If applicable, Number of Eggs Aspirated/Embryos Implanted/Location Implanted	Comments
_____	❑ AI	❑ IUI	_____	_____
_____	❑ GIFT	❑ ZIFT	_____	_____
_____	❑ IVF	❑ other	_____	_____
_____	❑ AI	❑ IUI	_____	_____
_____	❑ GIFT	❑ ZIFT	_____	_____
_____	❑ IVF	❑ other	_____	_____
_____	❑ AI	❑ IUI	_____	_____
_____	❑ GIFT	❑ ZIFT	_____	_____
_____	❑ IVF	❑ other	_____	_____
_____	❑ AI	❑ IUI	_____	_____
_____	❑ GIFT	❑ ZIFT	_____	_____
_____	❑ IVF	❑ other	_____	_____
_____	❑ AI	❑ IUI	_____	_____
_____	❑ GIFT	❑ ZIFT	_____	_____
_____	❑ IVF	❑ other	_____	_____
_____	❑ AI	❑ IUI	_____	_____
_____	❑ GIFT	❑ ZIFT	_____	_____
_____	❑ IVF	❑ other	_____	_____
_____			_____	_____

AI = artificial insemination; IUI = intrauterine insemination; GIFT = gamete intrafollopian transfer; ZIFT = zygote intrafallopian transfer; IVF = in vitro fertilization

Pregnancy Test Results

Pregnancy tests are simultaneously the most hopeful and scariest of tests. We hope that they are positive and dread that they are negative. But while potentially stressful, they are very necessary. A positive test can provide you with joy and the beginning of a healthy pregnancy. A negative test can resolve your month's quest and allow you to start trying again. But pregnancy tests can be very important for a third reason: monitoring for ectopic pregnancy is possible with pregnancy tests. Ectopic pregnancies occur when the embryo implants and starts to grow someplace outside of the proper spot within the uterus; the most common place is the fallopian tube. Even though it is outside of the uterus, the embryo continues to grow and it does not take long until it ruptures the tissues surrounding its location. When it ruptures, life-threatening hemorrhage can result. Ectopic pregnancies can jeopardize fertility and they are the leading cause of first trimester maternal death. Do you feel any abdominal or back pain? Unusual bleeding? Shoulder pain? Weakness? Dizziness? Don't wait: call your physician right away. Every time you take a pregnancy test—either a urine or a blood test—track the results here.

Pregnancy Test Results

Date	Type of Pregnancy Test	Results	Comments
	❑ urine (home)		
	❑ urine (lab)		
	❑ blood (qualitative)		
	❑ blood (quantitative)		
	❑ urine (home)		
	❑ urine (lab)		
	❑ blood (qualitative)		
	❑ blood (quantitative)		
	❑ urine (home)		
	❑ urine (lab)		
	❑ blood (qualitative)		
	❑ blood (quantitative)		
	❑ urine (home)		
	❑ urine (lab)		
	❑ blood (qualitative)		
	❑ blood (quantitative)		
	❑ urine (home)		
	❑ urine (lab)		
	❑ blood (qualitative)		
	❑ blood (quantitative)		

Pregnancy Test Results

Date	Type of Pregnancy Test	Results	Comments
	❑ urine (home)		
	❑ urine (lab)		
	❑ blood (qualitative)		
	❑ blood (quantitative)		
	❑ urine (home)		
	❑ urine (lab)		
	❑ blood (qualitative)		
	❑ blood (quantitative)		
	❑ urine (home)		
	❑ urine (lab)		
	❑ blood (qualitative)		
	❑ blood (quantitative)		
	❑ urine (home)		
	❑ urine (lab)		
	❑ blood (qualitative)		
	❑ blood (quantitative)		
	❑ urine (home)		
	❑ urine (lab)		
	❑ blood (qualitative)		
	❑ blood (quantitative)		

Pregnancy Test Results

Date	Type of Pregnancy Test	Results	Comments
	❑ urine (home)		
	❑ urine (lab)		
	❑ blood (qualitative)		
	❑ blood (quantitative)		
	❑ urine (home)		
	❑ urine (lab)		
	❑ blood (qualitative)		
	❑ blood (quantitative)		
	❑ urine (home)		
	❑ urine (lab)		
	❑ blood (qualitative)		
	❑ blood (quantitative)		
	❑ urine (home)		
	❑ urine (lab)		
	❑ blood (qualitative)		
	❑ blood (quantitative)		
	❑ urine (home)		
	❑ urine (lab)		
	❑ blood (qualitative)		
	❑ blood (quantitative)		

Pregnancy Test Results

Date	Type of Pregnancy Test	Results	Comments
	❏ urine (home)		
	❏ urine (lab)		
	❏ blood (qualitative)		
	❏ blood (quantitative)		
	❏ urine (home)		
	❏ urine (lab)		
	❏ blood (qualitative)		
	❏ blood (quantitative)		
	❏ urine (home)		
	❏ urine (lab)		
	❏ blood (qualitative)		
	❏ blood (quantitative)		
	❏ urine (home)		
	❏ urine (lab)		
	❏ blood (qualitative)		
	❏ blood (quantitative)		
	❏ urine (home)		
	❏ urine (lab)		
	❏ blood (qualitative)		
	❏ blood (quantitative)		

Pregnancy Test Results

Date	Type of Pregnancy Test	Results	Comments
	❑ urine (home)		
	❑ urine (lab)		
	❑ blood (qualitative)		
	❑ blood (quantitative)		
	❑ urine (home)		
	❑ urine (lab)		
	❑ blood (qualitative)		
	❑ blood (quantitative)		
	❑ urine (home)		
	❑ urine (lab)		
	❑ blood (qualitative)		
	❑ blood (quantitative)		
	❑ urine (home)		
	❑ urine (lab)		
	❑ blood (qualitative)		
	❑ blood (quantitative)		
	❑ urine (home)		
	❑ urine (lab)		
	❑ blood (qualitative)		
	❑ blood (quantitative)		

Pregnancy Test Results

Date	Type of Pregnancy Test	Results	Comments
_____	❑ urine (home)	_____	_____
_____	❑ urine (lab)	_____	_____
_____	❑ blood (qualitative)	_____	_____
_____	❑ blood (quantitative)	_____	_____
_____	❑ urine (home)	_____	_____
_____	❑ urine (lab)	_____	_____
_____	❑ blood (qualitative)	_____	_____
_____	❑ blood (quantitative)	_____	_____
_____	❑ urine (home)	_____	_____
_____	❑ urine (lab)	_____	_____
_____	❑ blood (qualitative)	_____	_____
_____	❑ blood (quantitative)	_____	_____
_____	❑ urine (home)	_____	_____
_____	❑ urine (lab)	_____	_____
_____	❑ blood (qualitative)	_____	_____
_____	❑ blood (quantitative)	_____	_____
_____	❑ urine (home)	_____	_____
_____	❑ urine (lab)	_____	_____
_____	❑ blood (qualitative)	_____	_____
_____	❑ blood (quantitative)	_____	_____
_____	_____	_____	_____

Pregnancy Test Results

Date	Type of Pregnancy Test	Results	Comments
	❑ urine (home)		
	❑ urine (lab)		
	❑ blood (qualitative)		
	❑ blood (quantitative)		
	❑ urine (home)		
	❑ urine (lab)		
	❑ blood (qualitative)		
	❑ blood (quantitative)		
	❑ urine (home)		
	❑ urine (lab)		
	❑ blood (qualitative)		
	❑ blood (quantitative)		
	❑ urine (home)		
	❑ urine (lab)		
	❑ blood (qualitative)		
	❑ blood (quantitative)		
	❑ urine (home)		
	❑ urine (lab)		
	❑ blood (qualitative)		
	❑ blood (quantitative)		

Your Personal Conception Plan

If you were traveling across country, chances are that you would develop some sort of plan; a roadmap to guide you to the destination of your choice. Even if you were free-spiritedly sowing wild oats on a trip across Europe or Asia, you would likely know if you were going east, west, north, or south. Without some direction, reaching a destination is nearly impossible. Use this section to sketch out your plan for becoming pregnant. It might start out "Go to an infertility specialist; find out what our obstacle to pregnancy is; resolve" and then become more specific, such as, "Take clomiphene at the low dose for three cycles; reevaluate if not pregnant." This plan may be done alone, with your partner, or in conjunction with your physician. Do you need some time off from the whole thing? It's perfectly reasonable to schedule yourself a "vacation" in this section, too.

One thing common to many women undergoing infertility treatment is the gradual, even unwitting, introduction to advanced medical technology. One moment we are healthy women trying to do the most natural thing in the world: get pregnant. The next, we are having an array of tests. Then we might start taking infertility medications. From there, it is easy to begin undertaking more and more complex procedures as we try to get pregnant. During this process, we often live two weeks "on" and two weeks "off." We prepare ourselves to conceive emotionally and medically (often with different treatments) during the first two weeks of each cycle; during the second two weeks we rest, take it easy, and push the idea of infertility aside while we imagine a growing embryo. This cyclic nature of infertility treatment can make it difficult to maintain a sense of the long term goal—a baby. We may get lost in the cycle, which can turn rather vicious. This is where the personal conception plan can help: developing your own plan and articulating exactly what your intermediate goals are can give direction to your efforts. For some women, however, the thought of writing down a plan may be burdensome, in which case it is perfectly all right to skip this section! It is here for you if you decide to use it in the future.

To help you get started, there are some sample entries. If you choose to write your plan down, remember that you are not married to any one idea; expect that your personal conception plan will have many incarnations! Feel free to erase, cross out, and start anew without worrying about neatness. This is your organizer—your journey—and no one will be grading your work. The personal conception plan is just that: personal. Its purpose is to assist you in organizing your thoughts about what you want to do—and what you do not; which steps you wish to take—and which you do not. (For me, this type of planning is absolutely necessary. Recently, it helped me know when to stop trying to get pregnant so intensely, and rest a bit. I was not ready for the economic or, more importantly, psychological impact of infertility treatment. Had I not taken the time to make my own plan, I would have gone full speed ahead with the program when I should have rested instead). Making your own plan gives you a chance to consider your course of action and your timeline, and will help make the most of any treatments you decide to undertake.

Your Personal Conception Plan

Sample

Goal	Target Date	If Has Not Occurred by Target Date Consider Next
Natural pregnancy with take-home baby	*1/1/99*	*ovulation induction with clomiphene citrate but no hCG shot*

Comments

Use all natural resources——temperature charting, ovulation predictor kits, etc., to time intercourse accurately——work with fertility doctor to be sure my husband and I are healthy with no obvious obstacles to pregnancy.

Goal	Target Date	If Has Not Occurred by Target Date Consider Next
Pregnancy with take-home baby using medicines to assist cycles	*7/1/99 (five or six cycles)*	*ovulation induction with clomiphene citrate, hCG shot, and IUI*

Comments

Watch ovulation closely with fertility doctor. How to schedule MD appointments with work? Check with supervisor about scheduling appointments during lunch breaks.

Comments

Comments

Your Personal Conception Plan

Goal	Target Date	If Has Not Occurred by Target Date Consider Next
_____	_____	_____
_____	_____	_____
_____	_____	_____

Comments _____

_____

_____

Goal	Target Date	If Has Not Occurred
_____	_____	_____
_____	_____	_____
_____	_____	_____

Comments _____

_____

_____

Goal	Target Date	If Has Not Occurred
_____	_____	_____
_____	_____	_____
_____	_____	_____

Comments _____

_____

Your Personal Conception Plan

Goal	Target Date	If Has Not Occurred by Target Date Consider Next
_____	_____	_____
_____	_____	_____
_____	_____	_____
_____	_____	_____

Comments _____

_____

_____

_____

| _____ | _____ | _____ |
| _____ | _____ | _____ |

Comments _____

_____

_____

_____

| _____ | _____ | _____ |
| _____ | _____ | _____ |

Comments _____

_____

_____

_____

_____	_____	_____
_____	_____	_____
_____	_____	_____

Comments _____

_____

Your Personal Conception Plan

Goal	Target Date	If Has Not Occurred by Target Date Consider Next
_____	_____	_____
_____	_____	_____
_____	_____	_____
_____	_____	_____

Comments _____

_____

_____

_____

| _____ | _____ | _____ |
| _____ | _____ | _____ |

Comments _____

_____

_____

| _____ | _____ | _____ |
| _____ | _____ | _____ |

Comments _____

_____

_____

| _____ | _____ | _____ |
| _____ | _____ | _____ |

Comments _____

_____

Your Personal Conception Plan

Goal	Target Date	If Has Not Occurred by Target Date Consider Next
_____	_____	_____
_____	_____	_____
_____	_____	_____

Comments _____

_____

_____

_____	_____	_____
_____	_____	_____
_____	_____	_____

Comments _____

_____

_____

_____	_____	_____
_____	_____	_____
_____	_____	_____

Comments _____

_____

Your Personal Conception Plan

Goal	Target Date	If Has Not Occurred by Target Date Consider Next
_____	_____	_____
_____	_____	_____
_____	_____	_____
_____	_____	_____

Comments _____

_____

_____

| _____ | _____ | _____ |
| _____ | _____ | _____ |

Comments _____

_____

_____

| _____ | _____ | _____ |
| _____ | _____ | _____ |

Comments _____

_____

_____

_____	_____	_____
_____	_____	_____
_____	_____	_____

Comments _____

_____

Your Medical History

There is nothing worse than forgetting when a key medical event occurred. This chart will allow you to track your and your partner's major medical events, as well as significant family medical information. Add each new event to this chart and you will have a permanent record of your essential medical information. Show this to your infertility specialist, too; perhaps seeing an event in your medical history will give him or her a clue to your infertility diagnosis. And when you pay a visit to a new physician—even if the visit is not related to your fertility—take this with you. A copy can go into your medical record, saving you from having to repeat this information.

Your Medical History (Female Partner)

General Medical History

	Date	Comments	Hospital/Health Care Provider
Significant Illnesses			
1.			
2.			
3.			
4.			
5.			
6.			
Surgeries			
1.			
2.			
3.			
4.			
5.			
6.			

Obstetrical/Gynecological History

Age of First Menstrual Period

Description of Menstrual Periods (e.g., mild cramping, heavy flow, etc.)

Contraceptive History (type and duration of contraceptives used)

Date Started Attempting Pregnancy

Past Pregnancies

1.

2.

Your Medical History (Female Partner, continued)

	Date	Comments	Hospital/Health Care Provider
Past Pregnancies			
3.			
4.			
5.			
6.			
Pre-Term Deliveries			
1.			
2.			
3.			
4.			
5.			
6.			
Miscarriages			
1.			
2.			
3.			
4.			
5.			
6.			
Ectopic Pregnancies			
1.			
2.			
3.			
4.			
5.			
6.			

Your Medical History (Female Partner, continued)

	Date	Comments	Hospital/Health Care Provider
Terminations			
1.			
2.			
3.			
4.			
5.			
6.			
Molar Pregnancies			
1.			
2.			
3.			
4.			
5.			
6.			
Abnormal Pap Smears/Treatments			
1.			
2.			
3.			
4.			
5.			
6.			
Sexually Transmitted Infections/Treatment			
1.			
2.			
3.			
4.			
5.			
6.			

Your Medical History (Female Partner, continued)

	Date	Comments	Hospital/Health Care Provider
Ovarian Cysts/Treatment			
1.			
2.			
3.			
4.			
5.			
6.			
Gynecologic Surgeries			
1.			
2.			
3.			
4.			
5.			
6.			

Significant Family Medical History

Mother			
Father			
Maternal Grandmother			
Maternal Grandfather			
Paternal Grandmother			
Paternal Grandfather			
Siblings			
1.			
2.			
3.			
4.			
5.			
6.			

Your Medical History (Female Partner, continued)

	Date	Comments	Hospital/Health Care Provider

Significant Obstetric/Gynecologic History of Mother, Sisters, Grandmothers

_____

_____

_____

_____

Other Significant Family History

_____

_____

_____

_____

Other Information

_____

_____

_____

_____

_____

_____

_____

_____

_____

_____

_____

_____

Your Medical History (Male Partner)

General Medical History

	Date	Comments	Hospital/Health Care Provider
Significant Illnesses			
1.			
2.			
3.			
4.			
5.			
6.			
Surgeries			
1.			
2.			
3.			
4.			
5.			
6.			

Fertility History

Children Fathered			
1.			
2.			
3.			
4.			
5.			
6.			

Past Pregnancies Fathered

Pregnancies Carried to Term			
1.			
2.			

Your Medical History (Male Partner, continued)

	Date	Comments	Hospital/Health Care Provider
Pregnancies Carried to Term			
3.			
4.			
5.			
6.			
Pre-Term Deliveries			
1.			
2.			
3.			
4.			
5.			
6.			
Miscarriages			
1.			
2.			
3.			
4.			
5.			
6.			
Ectopic Pregnancies			
1.			
2.			
3.			
4.			
5.			
6.			
7.			

Your Medical History (Male Partner, continued)

	Date	Comments	Hospital/Health Care Provider
Terminations			
1.			
2.			
3.			
4.			
5.			
6.			
Molar Pregnancies			
1.			
2.			
3.			
4.			
5.			
6.			
Sexually Transmitted Infections/Treatment			
1.			
2.			
3.			
4.			
5.			
6.			
Congenital Anomalies/ Testicular Maldescent			
Urinary Tract Infections			
Varicocele			
Mumps			
Epididymitis			
Prostatitis			

Your Medical History (Male Partner, continued)

	Date	Comments	Hospital/Health Care Provider
Hernia Repair			
Injuries			
1.			
2.			
3.			
4.			
5.			
6.			
Surgeries			
1.			
2.			
3.			
4.			
5.			
6.			

Significant Family Medical History

Mother			
Father			
Maternal Grandmother			
Maternal Grandfather			
Paternal Grandmother			
Paternal Grandfather			
Siblings			
1.			
2.			
3.			
4.			
5.			

Your Medical History (Male Partner, continued)

	Date	Comments	Hospital/Health Care Provider
Siblings			
6.			
7.			
Other Significant Family History			

Other Information

Useful Information

The basics. It is surprising how frequently one has to call the physician. Or the insurance company. Or the clinic nurse. Or needs other numbers that are really useful but who wants them cluttering up the limited and personal lines of an address book? Take a minute to write down important frequently used numbers and information so it is all in one place when you call someone or when you are at an appointment.

Name(s) _____

Address _____

Phone Number _____

Work Phone Numbers _____

Emergency Contact Information _____

Emergency Contact Information _____

Primary Care Physician _____ Phone _____

Address _____

Nurse _____ Phone _____

OB/Gyn _____ Phone _____

Address _____

Nurse _____ Phone _____

Infertility Specialist _____ Phone _____

Address _____

Nurse _____ Phone _____

Other Physician _____ Phone _____

Address _____

Nurse _____ Phone _____

Other Physician _____ Phone _____

Address _____

Nurse _____ Phone _____

Other Physician _____ Phone _____

Address _____

Nurse _____ Phone _____

Hospital/Clinic Financial Service Contact _____ Phone _____

Address _____

_____

Primary Insurance Company _____ Phone _____

Member ID _____

Group ID _____

Address _____

_____

Insurance Contact _____ Phone _____

Secondary Insurance Company _____ Phone _____

Member ID _____

Group ID _____

Address _____

_____

Insurance Contact _____ Phone _____

Known Allergies _____

_____

_____

Other Information _____

_____

_____

PART THREE

Charts about Information

Finding the Right Physician

This section allows you to document your search for the right physician. Record here information from friends, books, and medical referral sources; note your impressions from interviews with different physicians and any research you have done on them. Selecting a physician is always hard, but it may be even harder when the physician you seek is an infertility specialist. Try not to be convinced by success statistics alone; there are many other things to consider. For instance, you and your partner need to get along with your physician and the office staff. You should feel comfortable in the office. Will your physician mind if you call in the middle of the night with a concern? Does he or she explain procedures in a way you can understand them? Is fertility the main focus or is the physician a general OB/Gyn? Does the office or clinic take your insurance? Is the physician willing to go to bat for you with the insurance company if needed? Will he or she continue to see you after you become pregnant? If so, for how long? What range of services are provided? Does his or her philosophy about infertility treatment blend with yours? If you have already found the perfect physician—congratulations! But if you have not yet, bear in mind that finding the right physician for you is essential to having a good fertility experience; do not give up until you've found the right one.

Finding the Right Physician

M.D. Name

Phone

Address

Referred by

Comments

Questions & Answers

M.D. Name

Phone

Address

Referred by

Comments

Questions & Answers

M.D. Name

Phone

Address

Referred by

Comments

Questions & Answers

Finding the Right Physician

M.D. Name

Phone

Address

Referred by

Comments

Questions & Answers

M.D. Name

Phone

Address

Referred by

Comments

Questions & Answers

M.D. Name

Phone

Address

Referred by

Comments

Questions & Answers

Finding the Right Physician

M.D. Name _____

Phone _____

Address _____

Referred by _____

Comments _____

Questions & Answers _____

_____

_____

_____

_____

M.D. Name _____

Phone _____

Address _____

Referred by _____

Comments _____

Questions & Answers _____

_____

_____

_____

M.D. Name _____

Phone _____

Address _____

Referred by _____

Comments _____

Questions & Answers _____

_____

_____

Finding the Right Physician

M.D. Name

Phone

Address

Referred by

Comments

Questions & Answers

M.D. Name

Phone

Address

Referred by

Comments

Questions & Answers

M.D. Name

Phone

Address

Referred by

Comments

Questions & Answers

Finding the Right Physician

M.D. Name

Phone

Address

Referred by

Comments

Questions & Answers

_____

_____

_____

M.D. Name

Phone

Address

Referred by

Comments

Questions & Answers

_____

_____

_____

M.D. Name

Phone

Address

Referred by

Comments

Questions & Answers

_____

_____

_____

Keeping Track of References and Resources

The science of infertility and reproductive endocrinology advances practically daily. As a trip to any bookstore or a look on the internet will tell you, there are hundreds of resources available to you about infertility. Keep track here of references—books, articles, and information from other sources—that you find useful. Record the date you found each reference, what most interested you about the information, and the citation so you can find it again if you want to.

In the References and Resources section at the back of the book, there is a listing of resources that can improve your understanding of infertility evaluation and treatment. Some of them are popular references and others are more technical—do not let that scare you off! Infertility research is so complex and rapidly advancing that it may be what you need to know is not yet in all infertility books; it may only be in the medical literature, particularly the up-to-date medical journals and books. You do not need to understand all the terminology to understand such literature, you just need to be willing to try. There are many good medical dictionaries available at bookstores; get one and take it with you to a medical library. The glossary in the back of this book can help, too, for quick and easy reference. See a word you don't understand? Look it up. Not only will you learn a great deal from the literature, but you will have access to the same research that your physician does, as well as some of the same vocabulary. Your physician can answer questions you have about what you read, and this topic of conversation is a great opportunity for collaboration between the two of you. You can also look at medical textbooks—they can be enormously helpful. If you do not have a medical library close by, you can do some research on the internet; many medical journals and texts are now on-line, allowing you to browse the literature from your own home. Become a fertility—*your fertility*—expert by using all of the resources available to you.

Keeping Track of References and Resources

Topic

Date Referenced

Author

Reference (e.g., journal or book name, publisher, volume, pages)

Comments

Topic

Date Referenced

Author

Reference

Comments

Topic

Date Referenced

Author

Reference

Comments

Topic

Date Referenced

Author

Reference

Comments

Keeping Track of References and Resources

Topic

Date Referenced

Author

Reference (e.g., journal or book name, publisher, volume, pages)

Comments

Topic

Date Referenced

Author

Reference

Comments

Topic

Date Referenced

Author

Reference

Comments

Topic

Date Referenced

Author

Reference

Comments

Keeping Track of References and Resources

Topic

Date Referenced

Author

Reference (e.g., journal or book name, publisher, volume, pages)

Comments

Topic

Date Referenced

Author

Reference

Comments

Topic

Date Referenced

Author

Reference

Comments

Topic

Date Referenced

Author

Reference

Comments

Keeping Track of References and Resources

Topic

Date Referenced

Author

Reference (e.g., journal or book name, publisher, volume, pages)

Comments

Topic

Date Referenced

Author

Reference

Comments

Topic

Date Referenced

Author

Reference

Comments

Topic

Date Referenced

Author

Reference

Comments

Keeping Track of References and Resources

Topic _____

Date Referenced _____

Author _____

Reference (e.g., journal or book name, publisher, volume, pages) ____

Comments _____

_____

_____

Topic _____

Date Referenced _____

Author _____

Reference _____

Comments _____

_____

_____

Topic _____

Date Referenced _____

Author _____

Reference _____

Comments _____

_____

_____

Topic _____

Date Referenced _____

Author _____

Reference _____

Comments _____

_____

_____

Keeping Track of References and Resources

Topic

Date Referenced

Author

Reference (e.g., journal or book name, publisher, volume, pages)

Comments

Topic

Date Referenced

Author

Reference

Comments

Topic

Date Referenced

Author

Reference

Comments

Topic

Date Referenced

Author

Reference

Comments

Keeping Track of References and Resources

Topic _____

Date Referenced _____

Author _____

Reference (e.g., journal or book name, publisher, volume, pages) _____

Comments _____

_____

_____

Topic _____

Date Referenced _____

Author _____

Reference _____

Comments _____

_____

_____

Topic _____

Date Referenced _____

Author _____

Reference _____

Comments _____

_____

_____

Topic _____

Date Referenced _____

Author _____

Reference _____

Comments _____

_____

_____

Keeping Track of References and Resources

Topic _____

Date Referenced _____

Author _____

Reference (e.g., journal or book name, publisher, volume, pages) _____

Comments _____

_____

_____

Topic _____

Date Referenced _____

Author _____

Reference _____

Comments _____

_____

_____

Topic _____

Date Referenced _____

Author _____

Reference _____

Comments _____

_____

_____

Topic _____

Date Referenced _____

Author _____

Reference _____

Comments _____

_____

_____

Question and Answer Log

It is terrible to wake up in the middle of the night with an important question to ask your physician or check out in a book, only to awake the next morning having forgotten it. You will almost certainly have many questions for your physician as you journey toward motherhood. Write down your questions and the answers you receive here. This section may be expanded to include questions to ask yourself or your partner—how you might feel about a given issue, a potential treatment, or other such questions. Use this log freely to explore in a Q&A format anything you wish.

Question and Answer Log

Date

Question

Answer

Comments

_____

_____

_____

_____

Date

Question

Answer

Comments

_____

_____

_____

_____

Question and Answer Log

Date

Question

Answer

Comments

Date

Question

Answer

Comments

Date

Question

Answer

Comments

Date

Question

Answer

Comments

Question and Answer Log

Date

Question

Answer

Comments

_____

_____

_____

Date

Question

Answer

Comments

_____

_____

_____

Date

Question

Answer

Comments

_____

_____

_____

Date

Question

Answer

Comments

_____

_____

_____

Question and Answer Log

Date _____

Question _____

Answer _____

Comments _____

_____

_____

Date _____

Question _____

Answer _____

Comments _____

_____

_____

Date _____

Question _____

Answer _____

Comments _____

_____

_____

Date _____

Question _____

Answer _____

Comments _____

_____

_____

Question and Answer Log

Date _____

Question _____

Answer _____

Comments _____

_____

_____

_____

Date _____

Question _____

Answer _____

Comments _____

_____

_____

_____

Date _____

Question _____

Answer _____

Comments _____

_____

_____

_____

Date _____

Question _____

Answer _____

Comments _____

_____

_____

_____

Question and Answer Log

Date

Question

Answer

Comments

Date

Question

Answer

Comments

Date

Question

Answer

Comments

Date

Question

Answer

Comments

Question and Answer Log

Date _____

Question _____

Answer _____

Comments _____

_____

_____

_____

Date _____

Question _____

Answer _____

Comments _____

_____

_____

_____

Date _____

Question _____

Answer _____

Comments _____

_____

_____

_____

Date _____

Question _____

Answer _____

Comments _____

_____

_____

_____

Question and Answer Log

Date _____

Question _____

Answer _____

Comments _____

_____

_____

_____

Date _____

Question _____

Answer _____

Comments _____

_____

_____

_____

Date _____

Question _____

Answer _____

Comments _____

_____

_____

_____

Date _____

Question _____

Answer _____

Comments _____

_____

_____

_____

Question and Answer Log

Date _____

Question _____

Answer _____

Comments _____

_____

_____

_____

Date _____

Question _____

Answer _____

Comments _____

_____

_____

_____

Date _____

Question _____

Answer _____

Comments _____

_____

_____

_____

Date _____

Question _____

Answer _____

Comments _____

_____

_____

_____

Question and Answer Log

Date _____

Question _____

Answer _____

Comments _____

_____

_____

_____

Date _____

Question _____

Answer _____

Comments _____

_____

_____

_____

Date _____

Question _____

Answer _____

Comments _____

_____

_____

_____

Date _____

Question _____

Answer _____

Comments _____

_____

_____

_____

Financial Information

We are fortunate in the United States to have access to technologically advanced medical resources for all facets of human health. Researchers in numerous fields improve our knowledge of the human body; they discover treatments for a variety of conditions continuously. However, the complexities of health care insurance and finances have developed at an equally accelerated rate. Not all infertility evaluations or treatments may be covered by your insurance. Hospital and clinic billing can be extremely confusing. One of the best ways to stay on top of the financial information related to your infertility evaluation and treatment is to keep good records. The pages here are for you to document your interactions with insurance companies and health care facilities about payment issues. Are you being billed for a procedure your insurance should have covered? Call the insurance company right away. Are you hoping to be reimbursed for a procedure? Have your physician write a letter. Keep copies. Find out what infertility evaluations and treatments mandate coverage in your state. Are you confused about a bill you received from the clinic? Call the clinic and ask them to explain the bill. On the following chart keep track of every interaction about financial issues. Every time you talk with someone, document with whom you spoke, the time and date of your conversation, what was discussed, what was resolved, what actions were planned, and what is to be done next if your problem is not resolved by a specific date. That way, if the problem is not resolved, you will be prepared with detailed notes about what had been previously discussed.

Financial Information

Date/Time _____

Financial Issue _____

I Spoke To _____

Resolution and Comments _____

_____

_____

Date/Time _____

Financial Issue _____

I Spoke To _____

Resolution and Comments _____

_____

_____

Date/Time _____

Financial Issue _____

I Spoke To _____

Resolution and Comments _____

_____

_____

Date/Time _____

Financial Issue _____

I Spoke To _____

Resolution and Comments _____

_____

_____

Financial Information

Date/Time _____

Financial Issue _____

I Spoke To _____

Resolution and Comments _____

_____

_____

_____

Date/Time _____

Financial Issue _____

I Spoke To _____

Resolution and Comments _____

_____

_____

_____

Date/Time _____

Financial Issue _____

I Spoke To _____

Resolution and Comments _____

_____

_____

_____

Date/Time _____

Financial Issue _____

I Spoke To _____

Resolution and Comments _____

_____

_____

_____

Financial Information

Date/Time
_____

Financial Issue
_____

I Spoke To
_____

Resolution and Comments
_____

_____

_____

_____

Date/Time
_____

Financial Issue
_____

I Spoke To
_____

Resolution and Comments
_____

_____

_____

_____

Date/Time
_____

Financial Issue
_____

I Spoke To
_____

Resolution and Comments
_____

_____

_____

_____

Date/Time
_____

Financial Issue
_____

I Spoke To
_____

Resolution and Comments
_____

_____

_____

_____

Financial Information

Date/Time

Financial Issue

I Spoke To

Resolution and Comments

_____

_____

_____

Date/Time

Financial Issue

I Spoke To

Resolution and Comments

_____

_____

_____

Date/Time

Financial Issue

I Spoke To

Resolution and Comments

_____

_____

_____

Date/Time

Financial Issue

I Spoke To

Resolution and Comments

_____

_____

_____

Financial Information

Date/Time _____

Financial Issue _____

I Spoke To _____

Resolution and Comments _____

_____

_____

_____

Date/Time _____

Financial Issue _____

I Spoke To _____

Resolution and Comments _____

_____

_____

_____

Date/Time _____

Financial Issue _____

I Spoke To _____

Resolution and Comments _____

_____

_____

_____

Date/Time _____

Financial Issue _____

I Spoke To _____

Resolution and Comments _____

_____

_____

_____

Financial Information

Date/Time

Financial Issue

I Spoke To

Resolution and Comments

Date/Time

Financial Issue

I Spoke To

Resolution and Comments

Date/Time

Financial Issue

I Spoke To

Resolution and Comments

Date/Time

Financial Issue

I Spoke To

Resolution and Comments

Financial Information

Date/Time _____

Financial Issue _____

I Spoke To _____

Resolution and Comments _____

_____

_____

_____

Date/Time _____

Financial Issue _____

I Spoke To _____

Resolution and Comments _____

_____

_____

_____

Date/Time _____

Financial Issue _____

I Spoke To _____

Resolution and Comments _____

_____

_____

_____

Date/Time _____

Financial Issue _____

I Spoke To _____

Resolution and Comments _____

_____

_____

_____

Financial Information

Date/Time

Financial Issue

I Spoke To

Resolution and Comments

Date/Time

Financial Issue

I Spoke To

Resolution and Comments

Date/Time

Financial Issue

I Spoke To

Resolution and Comments

Date/Time

Financial Issue

I Spoke To

Resolution and Comments

Financial Information

Date/Time

Financial Issue

I Spoke To

Resolution and Comments

Date/Time

Financial Issue

I Spoke To

Resolution and Comments

Date/Time

Financial Issue

I Spoke To

Resolution and Comments

Date/Time

Financial Issue

I Spoke To

Resolution and Comments

Financial Information

Date/Time

Financial Issue

I Spoke To

Resolution and Comments

Date/Time

Financial Issue

I Spoke To

Resolution and Comments

Date/Time

Financial Issue

I Spoke To

Resolution and Comments

Date/Time

Financial Issue

I Spoke To

Resolution and Comments

Blank Pages for Notes

Here are some blank pages for you to write down notes about anything and everything. If you are talking with your physician and do not have sufficient time to put information in its proper chart, feel free to write it all down here and transfer it later. Other ideas, thoughts, feelings, or notes may be written here in a free-form fashion.

_____

_____

_____

_____

_____

_____

_____

_____

_____

_____

_____

_____

_____

_____

_____

_____

_____

_____

_____

_____

_____

PART FOUR

Once You Are Pregnant

Hopefully, you will become pregnant! The main goal of this section is to help you track information about your pregnancy in the same way you tracked information about your fertility. We'll also discuss some of the tools your physician might use to check on your pregnancy. Especially for the woman undergoing infertility treatment, fertility and pregnancy are on a continuum; as you go from trying to get pregnant to being pregnant, you will often see the same physician (at least for a little while) and you may have many of the same tests performed. Here you are provided with a means to track results from tests you have performed throughout those precious nine months. Keeping track of your pregnancy information will foster another collaborative relationship with your obstetrician. If you start seeing a new physician after you are pregnant, the fertility charts in the previous sections will make it easier to share pertinent information about your infertility evaluation and treatment. Don't forget: you should discuss everything—all of your questions, concerns, problems, everything—with your physician, just as you did during your infertility treatment.

Tools to Monitor Your Early Pregnancy

Infertility specialists differ in how long they will work with you after you become pregnant; some stay with you for at most the first eight weeks of pregnancy and others will deliver your baby. Ask your physician about his or her policy. If you will start seeing a new obstetrician during your pregnancy, your infertility specialist might be able to recommend one if you do not have one already.

There are many tools available to monitor your pregnancy and check on your baby's health status. Here are a few that may be used early on:

1. Ultrasound. Just as you may have had ultrasound performed during your infertility evaluation and treatment, you will probably have at least one ultrasound during your pregnancy. Early in the pregnancy, ultrasound allows measurement of your baby, which gives a good estimation of its gestational age. Depending on the age of the baby, your physician may look for a heartbeat. Once a heartbeat is detected, your chances of a miscarriage decrease dramatically. In fact, some infertility specialists use the presence of a heartbeat as the indication that it is time for you to move on to an obstetrician! Ultrasound may be used again later in pregnancy to check on your baby's growth, development, health status, and the placenta's implantation and functioning.

2. Tests of hormone levels. Hormones remain as important when you are pregnant as they were while you were trying to get pregnant. Because of this, you may have blood tests taken to measure hormone levels, particularly progesterone. Progesterone is essential to pregnancy: it quiets the uterus and keeps it from contracting. If you do not have enough, supplements may be recommended.

3. Other blood tests. At the beginning of your infertility evaluation, some infertility specialists run a series of tests in anticipation of your becoming pregnant. If not, your physician will as soon as you become pregnant. This series might include tests to measure your blood's oxygen-carrying capacity (hemoglobin and hematocrit), your blood type, presence of infections that can be passed to your baby, and your immunity to infections (such as rubella, which can be harmful to your baby if contracted during early pregnancy).

Other routinely performed tests during pregnancy are listed in the glossary. Pregnancy books contain detailed information about these tests, and your physician will be able to provide you with more information and answer any questions you have.

Preventing Miscarriage and Pre-Term Labor: Tracking Your Healthy Pregnancy

When I became pregnant, I was not aware that there was potential for difficulty ahead. Though I knew some women had miscarriages and difficult pregnancies, I thought such complications were very rare. I assumed most women had healthy, problem-free pregnancy experiences, emerging from nine months of bliss with a lovely infant in their arms. I was not aware that as many as 15 percent of clinically recognized pregnancies (that is, when a woman has a positive pregnancy test or a positive ultrasound) end in miscarriage (also known as spontaneous abortion). Pre-term labor occurs in as many as 10 percent of births and is a major cause of infant illness, injury, and mortality. It is natural to want to focus only on the positive: at last we're pregnant! Who wants to think about scary things such as miscarriage and pre-term labor, especially when most of the time the outcome will be positive? But if you are aware of signs and symptoms of potential problems from the beginning, you increase your chances of preventing miscarriage and pre-term labor. This is especially important because, as women with a history of infertility, we are at greater risk for these hazards. This section is not meant to alarm you—chances are very good that your pregnancy will be absolutely fine! The purpose of this section is to arm you with information to increase those chances for a positive outcome.

Possible Causes of Miscarriage

There are a number of causes of miscarriage. There are genetic factors in which, for a variety of reasons, the embryo's chromosomal composition is not compatible with life. While miscarriages due to chromosomal abnormalities can occur throughout the nine month period, they are most likely to occur during the first trimester. Some references indicate that as many as 60 percent of miscarriages that take place within the first trimester are chromosome-related. Anatomic factors in the mother—how her uterus or pelvic organs are formed, or how they have been affected by surgery or infection—can result in miscarriage as well. Hormonal factors, such as progesterone insufficiency, thyroid disorders, or diabetes, can cause miscarriage, as can disease in the mother, such as bacterial or viral illnesses, and cardiac, blood, or immune disorders. Finally, there are behavioral factors (like smoking, drinking, drugs) and environmental factors (like exposure to pollutants or toxins) that can sometimes lead to miscarriage.

It is rather frightening how many things can lead to problems in pregnancy. But before you panic, please recognize that these are not absolute causal factors: some women have risk factors for miscarriage but deliver healthy babies without any problems at all. The point is to be aware that miscarriages do happen, and to know the signs and symptoms in advance. That way, if something unusual does occur, you are prepared and can take action by seeing your physician immediately. If a problem is brewing, the earlier you seek medical assistance the higher the chance that the problem can be corrected.

Possible Causes of Pre-Term Labor

An infant is considered to be premature if his gestational age is less than 37 weeks or his birthweight is less than 2500 grams (about 5.5 pounds). There are multiple risk factors for pre-term labor and some of them parallel causes of miscarriage: anatomic factors in the mother, hormonal factors, and maternal disease. Placental abnormalities—when the baby's placental lifeline is either implanted incorrectly or malfunctioning—can be another cause of pre-term labor. Life-style factors such as smoking, drug use, inadequate weight gain, and inadequate prenatal care are other potentially alterable risk factors for pre-term labor. Interestingly, women who have had prior episodes of pre-term labor are at increased risk of future episodes.

Signs and Symptoms of Miscarriage and Pre-Term Labor

Each day a baby stays in its mother's womb is a big step toward its healthy beginning. To keep your baby tucked cozily inside you and promote its healthiest possible start to life, it is essential that you are aware of the signs of a possible problem. That way, if you see a sign, you can get help as soon as possible. Ask your physician in advance so you are familiar with warning signs of miscarriage and pre-term labor. Have them in your consciousness, not to scare yourself, but to be alert to them. If any of the symptoms occur, do not waste time: call your physician or go to the emergency room immediately.

Here are some signs of miscarriage and pre-term labor throughout pregnancy (in no particular order):

- increase or change in vaginal discharge (any change may be relevant, including if it looks sort of like mid-cycle cervical mucus ["highways for sperm"] did before you were pregnant);
- uterine contractions (may be mild, may even feel like your menstrual period used to);
- vaginal bleeding (may be spotting or frank bleeding);
- fluid leaking from vagina (may be all at once or a trickle);
- feeling of pelvic pressure, fullness, or congestion;
- backache or back pressure;

- diarrhea, urge to go to the bathroom, or intestinal pain (hormones that influence uterine contractions also impact the intestines);
- sense something is "wrong";
- continuous or episodic abdominal pain (may be sharp, dull, or achy);
- feeling sick, nauseated, or vomiting excessively;
- chills or fever;
- any other signs or symptoms your physician mentions to you.

Here are some signs of pre-term labor specific to the last three months of pregnancy (these are in addition to the above):
- any change in your baby's established pattern of activity;
- more than three contractions in an hour.

If you do have symptoms of a possible problem, it is natural to experience a sense of denial: "I'm just imagining this; everything's okay." While this may be useful to help you stay calm—which is good—do not let it dissuade you from seeking medical attention. If you have any symptoms of a possible problem with your pregnancy, do not delay: seek medical attention immediately. Call your physician or go to the emergency room right away. Do not worry if your concern turns out to be a "false alarm"—health care providers are available around the clock to help you and your growing baby, so you never need to be embarrassed about asking for their assistance.

If you experience any of the warning signs listed above or that your physician told you to be alert to, your physician will probably want to see what is going on. He or she may do blood work to check your hormone levels, do an ultrasound to check your baby in the uterus, do a physical exam to check your cervix, use a fetal monitor to listen to your baby's heartbeat, or check your uterine contractions—a number of tools are available to assess your baby's health status.

If there is a problem, we are fortunate to have several options to prevent miscarriage and slow or halt pre-term labor. Several of the books in the References and Resources section contain excellent information about miscarriage and pre-term labor prevention. Depending on your situation, your physician may recommend medications, procedures, or a combination of the two to help keep your baby in your womb until he or she is developed enough to be safely delivered.

Tracking Your Healthy Pregnancy

Throughout your pregnancy, you will have many routine tests performed. You may have blood work to check on your blood's oxygen-carrying capacity, an alpha-fetoprotein (AFP) test to screen for neural tube defects and Down syndrome, a test to see what blood type you are, hCG levels, and hormone measurements. Ultrasound monitoring and other tests (such as tests to check for the effect of contractions on the baby) may be performed to check for fetal well-being. Amniocentesis or chorionic villus sampling may be used to obtain the fetus' genetic information. Your physician may check your blood pressure, vital signs, weight, your body's ability to metabolize sugar in the bloodstream, and use other tests to check your health and the health of your growing baby. Two charts are available to track these routine evaluations: one on which to track the test results during your pregnancy and the other on which to track your weight and blood pressure at each obstetrical visit.

A third chart is available for your to keep a written record of your baby's movement, once you are able to feel your baby moving. Not only is it fun to take note of the baby's activity pattern—what does he or she do after you have eaten? when you are resting?—this written record can be useful as a source of comparison. Sudden changes or decreases in your baby's activity may represent only that his or her daily routine has changed, but they can also be early signals of a complication. Having a written record of the baby's usual activity pattern makes it easy to pinpoint precise differences in behavior. If you notice such changes, be sure to call your obstetrician right away.

Diagnostic Tests

Date/ Gestational Age	Test Name	Results	Comments
		❏ normal ❏ abnormal	
		❏ indeterminate	
		Specific result	
		❏ normal ❏ abnormal	
		❏ indeterminate	
		Specific result	
		❏ normal ❏ abnormal	
		❏ indeterminate	
		Specific result	
		❏ normal ❏ abnormal	
		❏ indeterminate	
		Specific result	

Diagnostic Tests

Date/ Gestational Age	Test Name	Results	Comments
		❏ normal ❏ abnormal	
		❏ indeterminate	
		Specific result	
		❏ normal ❏ abnormal	
		❏ indeterminate	
		Specific result	
		❏ normal ❏ abnormal	
		❏ indeterminate	
		Specific result	
		❏ normal ❏ abnormal	
		❏ indeterminate	
		Specific result	
		❏ normal ❏ abnormal	
		❏ indeterminate	
		Specific result	

Diagnostic Tests

Date/ Gestational Age	Test Name	Results	Comments
		❏ normal ❏ abnormal	
		❏ indeterminate	
		Specific result	
		❏ normal ❏ abnormal	
		❏ indeterminate	
		Specific result	
		❏ normal ❏ abnormal	
		❏ indeterminate	
		Specific result	
		❏ normal ❏ abnormal	
		❏ indeterminate	
		Specific result	
		❏ normal ❏ abnormal	
		❏ indeterminate	
		Specific result	
		❏ normal ❏ abnormal	
		❏ indeterminate	
		Specific result	

Diagnostic Tests

Date/ Gestational Age	Test Name	Results	Comments
		❑ normal ❑ abnormal ❑ indeterminate Specific result	
		❑ normal ❑ abnormal ❑ indeterminate Specific result	
		❑ normal ❑ abnormal ❑ indeterminate Specific result	
		❑ normal ❑ abnormal ❑ indeterminate Specific result	
		❑ normal ❑ abnormal ❑ indeterminate Specific result	
		❑ normal ❑ abnormal ❑ indeterminate Specific result	

Diagnostic Tests

Date/ Gestational Age	Test Name	Results	Comments
		❑ normal ❑ abnormal	
		❑ indeterminate	
		Specific result	
		❑ normal ❑ abnormal	
		❑ indeterminate	
		Specific result	
		❑ normal ❑ abnormal	
		❑ indeterminate	
		Specific result	
		❑ normal ❑ abnormal	
		❑ indeterminate	
		Specific result	
		❑ normal ❑ abnormal	
		❑ indeterminate	
		Specific result	
		❑ normal ❑ abnormal	
		❑ indeterminate	
		Specific result	

Diagnostic Tests

Date/ Gestational Age	Test Name	Results	Comments
		❏ normal ❏ abnormal	
		❏ indeterminate	
		Specific result	
		❏ normal ❏ abnormal	
		❏ indeterminate	
		Specific result	
		❏ normal ❏ abnormal	
		❏ indeterminate	
		Specific result	
		❏ normal ❏ abnormal	
		❏ indeterminate	
		Specific result	
		❏ normal ❏ abnormal	
		❏ indeterminate	
		Specific result	
		❏ normal ❏ abnormal	
		❏ indeterminate	
		Specific result	

Diagnostic Tests

Date/ Gestational Age	Test Name	Results	Comments
		❏ normal ❏ abnormal	
		❏ indeterminate	
		Specific result	
		❏ normal ❏ abnormal	
		❏ indeterminate	
		Specific result	
		❏ normal ❏ abnormal	
		❏ indeterminate	
		Specific result	
		❏ normal ❏ abnormal	
		❏ indeterminate	
		Specific result	
		❏ normal ❏ abnormal	
		❏ indeterminate	
		Specific result	
		❏ normal ❏ abnormal	
		❏ indeterminate	
		Specific result	

Weight and Blood Pressure Tracking

Date/ Gestational Age	Weight	Blood Pressure	Comments
	❑ kg ❑ lbs	❑ normal ❑ abnormal	
		/ mm Hg	
		❑ right arm ❑ left arm	
		❑ lying ❑ sitting ❑ standing	
	❑ kg ❑ lbs	❑ normal ❑ abnormal	
		/ mm Hg	
		❑ right arm ❑ left arm	
		❑ lying ❑ sitting ❑ standing	
	❑ kg ❑ lbs	❑ normal ❑ abnormal	
		/ mm Hg	
		❑ right arm ❑ left arm	
		❑ lying ❑ sitting ❑ standing	
	❑ kg ❑ lbs	❑ normal ❑ abnormal	
		/ mm Hg	
		❑ right arm ❑ left arm	
		❑ lying ❑ sitting ❑ standing	
	❑ kg ❑ lbs	❑ normal ❑ abnormal	
		/ mm Hg	
		❑ right arm ❑ left arm	
		❑ lying ❑ sitting ❑ standing	

Weight and Blood Pressure Tracking

Date/ Gestational Age	Weight	Blood Pressure	Comments
	❑ kg ❑ lbs	❑ normal ❑ abnormal	
		/ mm Hg	
		❑ right arm ❑ left arm	
		❑ lying ❑ sitting ❑ standing	
	❑ kg ❑ lbs	❑ normal ❑ abnormal	
		/ mm Hg	
		❑ right arm ❑ left arm	
		❑ lying ❑ sitting ❑ standing	
	❑ kg ❑ lbs	❑ normal ❑ abnormal	
		/ mm Hg	
		❑ right arm ❑ left arm	
		❑ lying ❑ sitting ❑ standing	
	❑ kg ❑ lbs	❑ normal ❑ abnormal	
		/ mm Hg	
		❑ right arm ❑ left arm	
		❑ lying ❑ sitting ❑ standing	
	❑ kg ❑ lbs	❑ normal ❑ abnormal	
		/ mm Hg	
		❑ right arm ❑ left arm	
		❑ lying ❑ sitting ❑ standing	

Weight and Blood Pressure Tracking

Date/ Gestational Age	Weight	Blood Pressure	Comments
	❑ kg ❑ lbs	❑ normal ❑ abnormal	
		/ mm Hg	
		❑ right arm ❑ left arm	
		❑ lying ❑ sitting ❑ standing	
	❑ kg ❑ lbs	❑ normal ❑ abnormal	
		/ mm Hg	
		❑ right arm ❑ left arm	
		❑ lying ❑ sitting ❑ standing	
	❑ kg ❑ lbs	❑ normal ❑ abnormal	
		/ mm Hg	
		❑ right arm ❑ left arm	
		❑ lying ❑ sitting ❑ standing	
	❑ kg ❑ lbs	❑ normal ❑ abnormal	
		/ mm Hg	
		❑ right arm ❑ left arm	
		❑ lying ❑ sitting ❑ standing	
	❑ kg ❑ lbs	❑ normal ❑ abnormal	
		/ mm Hg	
		❑ right arm ❑ left arm	
		❑ lying ❑ sitting ❑ standing	

Weight and Blood Pressure Tracking

Date/ Gestational Age	Weight	Blood Pressure	Comments
	❑ kg ❑ lbs	❑ normal ❑ abnormal	
		/ mm Hg	
		❑ right arm ❑ left arm	
		❑ lying ❑ sitting ❑ standing	
	❑ kg ❑ lbs	❑ normal ❑ abnormal	
		/ mm Hg	
		❑ right arm ❑ left arm	
		❑ lying ❑ sitting ❑ standing	
	❑ kg ❑ lbs	❑ normal ❑ abnormal	
		/ mm Hg	
		❑ right arm ❑ left arm	
		❑ lying ❑ sitting ❑ standing	
	❑ kg ❑ lbs	❑ normal ❑ abnormal	
		/ mm Hg	
		❑ right arm ❑ left arm	
		❑ lying ❑ sitting ❑ standing	
	❑ kg ❑ lbs	❑ normal ❑ abnormal	
		/ mm Hg	
		❑ right arm ❑ left arm	
		❑ lying ❑ sitting ❑ standing	

Weight and Blood Pressure Tracking

Date/ Gestational Age	Weight	Blood Pressure	Comments
	❑ kg ❑ lbs	❑ normal ❑ abnormal	
		/ mm Hg	
		❑ right arm ❑ left arm	
		❑ lying ❑ sitting ❑ standing	
	❑ kg ❑ lbs	❑ normal ❑ abnormal	
		/ mm Hg	
		❑ right arm ❑ left arm	
		❑ lying ❑ sitting ❑ standing	
	❑ kg ❑ lbs	❑ normal ❑ abnormal	
		/ mm Hg	
		❑ right arm ❑ left arm	
		❑ lying ❑ sitting ❑ standing	
	❑ kg ❑ lbs	❑ normal ❑ abnormal	
		/ mm Hg	
		❑ right arm ❑ left arm	
		❑ lying ❑ sitting ❑ standing	
	❑ kg ❑ lbs	❑ normal ❑ abnormal	
		/ mm Hg	
		❑ right arm ❑ left arm	
		❑ lying ❑ sitting ❑ standing	

Fetal Activity Pattern

Date Charted/ Gestational Age	Morning Movement	Afternoon Movement	Movement in Relation to Evening Movement	Movement in Relation to Maternal Resting	Maternal Activity

Fetal Activity Pattern

Date Charted/ Gestational Age	Morning Movement	Afternoon Movement	Movement in Relation to Evening Movement	Movement in Relation to Maternal Resting	Maternal Activity

Fetal Activity Pattern

Date Charted/ Gestational Age	Morning Movement	Afternoon Movement	Movement in Relation to Evening Movement	Movement in Relation to Maternal Resting	Maternal Activity

Fetal Activity Pattern

Date Charted/ Gestational Age	Morning Movement	Afternoon Movement	Movement in Relation to Evening Movement	Movement in Relation to Maternal Resting	Maternal Activity

PART FIVE

A Final Word

There is much wisdom to be gained along your path to motherhood. The importance of the journey is not only the goals that lie ahead—pregnancy and a healthy baby—but the personal enrichment that the process itself has to offer. Even if the road is difficult at times, everything you experience while seeking pregnancy will bring you closer to your goals and to a deeper understanding of your body, yourself, and your relationships. As my husband and I have experienced our own obstacles, we have sometimes reflected on the fact that they have given us the opportunity to deeply consider what it is to be parents—why we want to have children, the environment in which we wish to raise them, and how we want to parent them; and this is an opportunity not everyone has. As you organize and document your efforts toward your goals, feel proud of your progress, for it is important and meaningful.

Best wishes to you for great luck and much fertility!

Glossary

ABORTION *Also known as miscarriage.* Medically, there are several types of abortion, all referring to termination of pregnancy before an embryo or fetus is viable. The types of abortion you are most likely to hear about include spontaneous abortion—termination of pregnancy with no evident cause; habitual abortion—three or more spontaneous abortions in a row; incomplete abortion—an abortion in which not all the products of conception leave the uterus on their own; and threatened abortion—when signs or symptoms occur that might indicate abortion, including bleeding, cramping, or pain. Threatened abortions may or may not progress to spontaneous abortion.

ADHESIONS Scar tissue that has formed due to infection, surgery, or another cause. If it is in the fallopian tube or the uterus, it may interfere with transport of sperm to the egg, blastocyst to the uterus, or implantation of the blastocyst into the uterine lining. Asherman's syndrome refers to scar tissue in the uterus caused by excessive scraping and irritation of the uterine lining during surgery (such as D&C), or, sometimes, by infection.

ADRENAL GLAND Triangular shaped glands that sit atop the kidneys. Part of the endocrine system, they release multiple hormones controlling major aspects of human physiology (e.g., blood pressure, heart function, breathing, energy modulation, etc.).

AGGLUTINATION Clumping together or adherence of surfaces.

ALPHA FETOPROTEIN TEST (AFP) A screening procedure using a sample of the mother's blood during the second trimester of pregnancy (usually around 16 weeks of gestation). This test can reveal the possibility of chromosomal disorders (like Down syndrome) and of neural tube defects (incorrect development of the fetus's nervous system). Because it is only a screening test, a positive test indicates further testing may be needed—like amniocentesis or CVS; it is not in itself a definitive diagnosis.

AMENORRHEA Absence of the menstrual periods; may be normal (as in before puberty, during pregnancy, after menopause) or a result of a variety of causes, including emotional stress, malnutrition, hormonal imbalance, etc. May be primary, as in a woman who is over 18 and has never menstruated, or secondary, as in cessation of menses in a woman who has already menstruated.

AMNIOCENTESIS A diagnostic procedure generally performed in the second trimester of pregnancy (usually between 14 and 20 weeks of gestation) to obtain a sample of amniotic fluid. The fluid is studied to see if there are any genetic disorders in the fetus; can also indicate fetus's gender. May also be performed in the later stages of pregnancy to estimate the maturation of the fetus's lung tissue. Performed by inserting a needle through the mother's abdomen into the amniotic sac and withdrawing a small amount of amniotic fluid.

ANDROGENS A category of hormone found in both males and females in differing amounts; includes testosterone. Androgen release is directed by the endocrine system.

ANOVULULAR CYCLE When a woman's menstrual cycle is not accompanied by maturation and release of an ovum.

ANTIBODIES The human immune system has two lines of defense against illnesses and foreign bodies: one is the cell-mediated, the other is the humoral. T-cells operate the cell-mediated arm of the immune defense, attacking invaders directly on a cell-to-cell basis, while B-cells (or plasma lymphocytes) operate the humoral. The humoral response involves production of antibodies in response to antigens, which exist on the surface of foreign cells. Antibodies are able to detect the shape of these antigens and then, rather like a puzzle piece, lock onto the antigen and attack it. Sometimes, for a variety of reasons (some known and many unknown), a person will produce antibodies to their own cells (auto-antibodies), to sperm (antisperm antibodies), or to a developing embryo; this may result in illness, infertility in males and females, or miscarriage.

ANTIGENS *See Antibodies.*

ANTISPERM ANTIBODIES *See Antibodies.*

ARTIFICIAL INSEMINATION (AI) A means of inserting sperm into the woman's reproductive system other than intercourse; in AI, sperm are inserted into the woman's vagina near her cervix. May be with the woman's partner's sperm (artificial insemination husband [AIH]) or with a donor's sperm (artificial insemination donor [AID]).

ASHERMAN'S SYNDROME *See Adhesions.*

ASSISTED REPRODUCTIVE TECHNOLOGY (ART) Types of procedures that can help an infertile or subfertile couple conceive a child, including in vitro fertilization (IVF), gamete intrafallopian transfer (GIFT), and zygote intrafallopian transfer (ZIFT).

ASTHENOSPERMIA Low sperm motility.

AUTO-ANTIBODIES *See Antibodies.*

AZOOSPERMIA Absence of sperm in semen.

BASAL BODY TEMPERATURE (BBT) The temperature taken before getting out of bed each morning (and before eating, drinking, or moving about too much). When charted carefully, BBT monitoring can reveal when a woman is ovulating and if her progesterone levels are about right. Some terms used in interpreting a BBT chart: Biphasic—If a woman's temperature rises with ovulation, her BBT chart will show two phases, one lower and one higher. Before ovulation the temperature will be about half to a whole degree lower than after ovulation. The proliferative stage corresponds to the time before the elevation when the uterine lining is built up under the direction of hormones including estrogen. After ovulation, the temperature increases under the influence of progesterone in what is called the secretory or luteal phase. During this second phase, progesterone (much of it from the corpus luteum) helps to make the uterine lining soft and prepared for the incoming embryo. Monophasic—If a woman's BBT chart shows no ovulatory increase in temperature it might be called monophasic. This may mean she did not ovulate during that cycle or that there was an error in her charting or temperature measurement. Some women do ovulate, however, and do not show a temperature increase even though everything may be perfectly normal.

BETA HCG TEST A very sensitive blood test able to detect early pregnancies and to evaluate embryonic development, through measurement of human chorionic gonadotropin (hCG). *See also hCG Test and Human Chorionic Gonadotropin.*

BIOPSY Sampling of a small piece of tissue for diagnostic purposes.

BIPHASIC *See Basal Body Temperature (BBT).*

BLASTOCYST Stage of very early embryo development, occurring at about the time the embryo implants in the uterine lining.

BRAXTON HICKS CONTRACTIONS Painless uterine contractions felt during pregnancy; Braxton Hicks contractions are one way the uterus prepares itself for labor.

CAPACITATION *See Sperm Washing.*

CERVICAL CERCLAGE *See Incompetent Cervix.*

CERVICAL MUCUS A fluid that protects the opening of the cervix and entry into the uterus. Keeps bacteria, viruses, and sperm from entering the uterus. Cervical mucus is under hormonal control; usually thick and pasty, at ovulation cervical mucus becomes like egg white—clear, stretchy, and slippery due to the influence of estrogen. This "highway for sperm" allows passage of the sperm into the uterus via the cervix and, en route, helps ready the sperm for the uterine environment. Cervical mucus assessment is useful in assessing time of ovulation, and is used in many sympto-thermal methods of conception and contraception. Terms related to cervical mucus assessment: ferning—response to estrogen in the system, which makes the mucus thin on a microscopic slide; spinnbarkeit—stretchiness of cervical mucus (should be very stretchy around ovulation); hostile mucus—when the mucus does not have these qualities to help sperm into the uterus.

CERVICAL STENOSIS Narrowing of the cervix due to a congenital defect or, sometimes, as a result of scarring from infection or surgery.

CERVIX The entrance to the uterus from the vagina, also known as the neck of the uterus. Made of connective tissue, the cervix remains closed until an infant is delivered. At the time of delivery, the cervix dilates (opens) to allow the baby to come out.

CHORION The tissue that surrounds the baby and connects to the endometrium, giving rise to the placenta.

CHORIONIC VILLUS SAMPLING (CVS) A diagnostic procedure generally performed in the first trimester of pregnancy (usually between 6 and 8 weeks of gestation) to obtain a sample of the cells that later become part of the placenta. The cells can be studied to see if there are any genetic disorders in the fetus; can also indicate fetus's gender. A tiny sample of the finger-like projections (villi) of the chorion are removed via a small catheter inserted either into the cervix or through the mother's abdomen.

CHROMOSOME The DNA-carrying component of each cell, lying within the cell's nucleus (vital center point of each cell). In human reproduction, the male contributes 23 chromosomes and the female contributes 23, resulting in a total of 46 chromosomes in each human cell that direct growth and development and transmit all necessary genetic material. Forty-four of each human's chromosomes are autosomes (non-sex chromosomes); the two remaining are sex chromosomes. Sperm may carry X or Y sex chromosomes; eggs always carry X. Males result from the merging of a Y sperm with an X egg (sometimes denoted XY); females result from the merging of an X sperm with an X egg (sometimes denoted XX). Division of autosomes and other cells in the body is called mitosis; specialized division of sex cells is called meiosis (special because it allows cells related to reproduction to have only 23 chromosomes each, so that when the sperm and egg combine, the resulting number is 46 and not 92).

CILIA Tiny hairlike processes that line the inside surface of many tissues, including lung tissue, nasal passages, and the fallopian tubes. In the fallopian tubes, the cilia make a wave-like movement that ushers the egg and the sperm-egg combination toward the uterus.

CLOMIPHENE CHALLENGE TEST A test performed to see if the ovaries are capable of hormonal stimulation and ovulation.

CONDOM THERAPY Somewhat controversial therapy designed to reduce a woman's antibody reaction to her partner's sperm (e.g., to reduce anti-sperm antibodies). A woman may be advised to have her partner use a condom for as many as six months to prevent her contact with his sperm.

CORPUS LUTEUM After ovulation, the follicle that released the egg becomes a progesterone-producing organ within the ovary. Its production of progesterone prepares the uterine lining (endometrium) for an incoming embryo. If the embryo's production of hCG signals it to continue production of progesterone, the corpus luteum continues to do so until the placenta is able to take over. Otherwise, it is pre-programmed to decompose about 10 to 14 days after ovulation, which allows the uterine lining to shed (the menstrual period), and the cycle to begin again.

CORPUS LUTEUM CYSTS Functional cysts that develop in a woman's ovaries out of the corpus luteum; almost always benign, they may be symptomatic or hemorrhagic, but generally dissolve on their own in concert with the woman's cycle.

CRYPTORCHIDISM (UNDESCENDED TESTICLES) A developmental problem in which the testicles of a male child do not descend from the abdominal cavity into the scrotum by one year of age. Generally requires surgical repair.

DES (DIETHYLSTILBESTROL) A medication used in the 1950s for the prevention of miscarriage. DES had teratogenic effects in some offspring of women who used the drug during their pregnancies, including clear cell vaginal adenocarcinoma (a very rare cancer) in females and structural anomalies of the reproductive organs of males and females.

DILATE To open or widen.

DILATION AND CURETTAGE (D&C) A medical procedure in which the cervix is dilated and the uterine contents scraped (curettage).

DONOR INSEMINATION *See Artificial Insemination.*

DOWN SYNDROME A chromosomal abnormality (also called trisomy 21) that produces moderate to severe mental retardation, along with a syndrome of other physical effects. Risk of bearing a child with Down Syndrome increases with a woman's age. Presence of this chromosomal anomaly may be confirmed before a baby is born with amniocentesis or CVS.

DYSMENORRHEA Pain with menstruation, may range from mild to severe and take a variety of forms.

ECTOPIC PREGNANCY (EP) A pregnancy that occurs anywhere outside of the proper location within the uterus. While EP may occur in the abdomen, the ovary, an inappropriate place in the uterus, or in between tissues, it usually occurs in the fallopian tube. EP is the major cause of maternal death in the first trimester, generally due to rupture of the organ of implantation and subsequent hemorrhage. EP also can cause infertility by blocking the affected organ (usually fallopian tube) with scar tissue, or through surgery necessary to remove the products of conception and control hemorrhage. Warning signs: missed period, pallor, unusual vaginal bleeding (even in the presence of a menstrual period), abdominal or back pain, dizziness, nausea, shoulder pain, or faintness. If you have any of these symptoms, contact your physician right away and get a pregnancy test, even if you think you could not possibly be pregnant or if you have a confirmed pregnancy.

EGG RETRIEVAL A procedure used to obtain eggs from ovarian follicles for ARTs (e.g., IVF, GIFT, ZIFT), surrogacy, or egg donation. Usually performed under anesthesia, a long needle guided by ultrasound aspirates the eggs (using a syringe with gentle suction); alternately, a small incision may be made and the eggs extracted through the abdomen.

EJACULATE The semen and sperm released during a male's ejaculation.

EMBRYO After the sperm and egg join, the cells multiply, turning into a blastocyst. The blastocyst implants in the uterine lining within a week after conception, and is called an embryo from the second to eighth weeks of gestation; from the third to the ninth month, it is called a fetus.

EMBRYO TRANSFER In ARTs, when sperm and egg are joined and allowed to fertilize in a laboratory, the resulting zygote is returned to the woman's uterus (in the case of IVF) or the fallopian tube (in the case of ZIFT) via embryo transfer.

ENDOCRINE SYSTEM A group of glands that have no ducts, and release hormones directly into the bloodstream. The hormones are circulated throughout the body, and target specific organs for hormonal action. Endocrine glands include the hypothalamus, pineal gland, pituitary, thyroid, parathyroid, remaining part of the thymus gland (decreases with maturation), adrenal glands, pancreas, ovary, and testis.

ENDOMETRIAL BIOPSY A diagnostic procedure sometimes used in the second half of the menstrual cycle to check for luteal phase defect or other problems with the uterine lining. A sample of the uterine lining is collected for analysis to see if ovulation has occurred and if the proper hormonal balance has been produced.

ENDOMETRIOSIS A condition in which the uterine lining (endometrium) implants outside of the uterus. Endometrial tissue may enter the abdominal cavity, the ovaries, or other inappropriate locations. The condition may be mild to severe, interfering with fertility as well as causing other complications.

ENDOMETRIUM The uterine lining.

EPIDIDYMIS A thin, coiled, tubular body connected to and lying atop each testicle. Important for finalization of sperm development, mature sperm swim from the epididymis through the vas deferens.

ESTROGENS Female sex hormones, either natural or artificial. Natural female sex hormones (may be referred to as simply "estrogens") include estradiol and estrone, both produced in the ovaries under direction of the endocrine system. Estriol is the result of metabolism of estrogens and is found in urine. Often measured in infertility treatment, estrogen levels reveal a great deal about the menstrual cycle and state of ovulation. Artificial estrogen may be given for medical reasons, including hormone difficulties resulting from menopause.

FALLOPIAN TUBES (ALSO KNOWN AS OVIDUCTS) Thin cilia-lined tubes, the fallopian tubes connect the uterus to the ovaries, one on each side of the uterus. Gentle petal-like projections called fimbria are at the ovary side of each tube, and help bring the ovulated egg into the tube, where it is gently pushed in the direction of the uterus. Fertilization occurs in the fallopian tubes.

FALLOPOSCOPY A procedure in which a fiber optic device is used to visualize the fallopian tubes. Can diagnose blockages and abnormalities.

FECUNDITY *See Infertility.*

FERNING *See Cervical Mucus.*

FERTILIZATION The union of a sperm and an egg; the combination of genetic material.

FETUS From the third to the ninth month of gestation the infant is called a fetus.

FIMBRIA *See Fallopian Tubes.*

FOLLICLE STIMULATING HORMONE (FSH) Hormone released by the pituitary in response to stimulus from the hypothalamus, causing sperm development in testis of males and follicle growth in ovaries of females.

FOLLICLES Egg-containing sacs in the ovaries.

FOLLICULAR FLUID The nutrient-rich fluid within each follicle; supports the developing egg until ovulation. The fluid released at ovulation may help the fimbria of the fallopian tubes better pull the egg into the oviduct.

GALACTORRHEA Discharge from breasts (either milky or clear); may be associated with elevated prolactin.

GAMETE A mature reproductive cell; eggs for females and sperm for males.

GAMETE INTRAFALLOPIAN TRANSFER (GIFT) An ART procedure that evolved from the IVF procedure. Following superovulation using medications under an infertility specialist's careful observation, eggs are aspirated (extracted with a very fine needle, usually while she is anesthetized) from a woman's ovaries. The resulting eggs are mixed with sperm (but not allowed to fertilize in the laboratory) and inserted into the woman's fallopian tubes (she must have at least one open tube for GIFT). Because this mimics natural fertilization in the tubes rather than in the uterus, the success rates are usually higher for GIFT than for IVF.

GESTATIONAL AGE The length of time from conception to the time the assessment is being made. Full term human gestation (the time from conception to birth) is considered from 37 to 41 weeks.

GONADOTROPIN RELEASING HORMONE (GNRH) Secreted by the hypothalamus, GnRH acts on the pituitary to cause release of the appropriate gonadotropic hormones, such as FSH and LH.

HAMSTER EGG TEST (ALSO KNOWN AS SPERM PENETRATION ASSAY OR SPA) A test of the ability of sperm to penetrate a hamster egg. Hypothetically reveals if sperm are able to fertilize a human egg, although some sperm fail this test but are capable of fertilizing a human egg anyway. No embryo results from this test.

HCG TEST May be either a urine or a blood test that measures the amount (quantitative) or the presence (qualitative) of human chorionic gonadotropin (hCG) in a woman's body by one of various methods. In addition to revealing if there is an embryo, quantitative hCG testing can yield a profile of embryonic development and health. *See also Beta hCG Test.*

HOSTILE MUCUS *See Cervical Mucus.*

HUMAN CHORIONIC GONADOTROPIN (HCG) Hormone produced in early pregnancy; necessary to keep corpus luteum producing progesterone and prevent shedding of the uterine lining. Also used to simulate LH surge in some infertility treatments and cause ovulation.

HYPER- prefix indicating too much of something, such as hyperglycemia, which is too much sugar in the blood.

HYPERPROLACTINEMIA Condition with several causes in which the pituitary gland releases too much of the hormone prolactin. May interfere with fertility.

HYPERSTIMULATION OF THE OVARIES (ALSO KNOWN AS OVARIAN HYPERSTIMULATION SYNDROME) When using medications to induce superovulation, a rare but potentially life-threatening situation can occur. With many follicles enlarged, ovaries enlarge, too. The fluid that fills the follicles is rich with estrogen; if the eggs are allowed to ovulate (e.g., with a shot of hCG to simulate the LH surge), all this estrogenic fluid pours into the pelvic and abdominal regions. Rising hormone levels cause fluid to accumulate inappropriately in tissues. The ovarian cysts can rupture and cause hemorrhage. When ARTs first started, this side effect was much more common; now that there is effective ultrasound monitoring and better understanding of the syndrome, serious cases are very rare. In cases with too many prepared follicles seen on ultrasound, the hCG shot can be withheld, preventing release of the estrogenic follicular fluid and circumventing the problem. The ovaries are given a chance to return to normal before trying again.

HYPO- prefix indicating too little of something, such as hypoglycemic, which is too little sugar in the blood.

HYPOTHALAMUS A significant organ of the endocrine system, the hypothalamus sits in the brain atop the pituitary. The hypothalamus directs the pituitary with GnRH to release LH and FSH, which stimulates most reproductive functions in both males and females.

HYSTEROSALPINGOGRAM (HSG) To assess malformations of a woman's pelvic region, including fallopian tube obstructions, a dye (usually iodine based) is inserted through the cervix. X-ray pictures are taken as the fluid flows through the uterus, the fallopian tubes, and out the fimbriated ends of the tubes toward the ovaries.

HYSTEROSCOPY To assess uterine abnormalities, a very small fiberoptic device is inserted into the uterus while the woman is under anesthesia. May be used as a diagnostic procedure or to correct small problems surgically.

IMPOTENCE The inability of a man to have or maintain an erection; may be physiologic, psychologic, or due to illness.

INCOMPETENT (OR WEAKENED) CERVIX A pregnant woman's cervix can open prematurely during her pregnancy, usually early in the second trimester, if weakened congenitally or due to prior procedures or surgery to the cervix. Cervical cerclage is a procedure used in cases of incompetent or weakened cervix to reinforce the cervix and prevent labor until the infant is full term: while under anesthesia, a woman's cervix is stitched closed with a drawstring-like suture. Around 37 weeks, the stitch is removed to allow passage of the infant.

INFERTILITY A common definition is the inability of a couple to conceive after a year of unprotected intercourse; impaired fecundity often refers to couples who are infertile by this same definition plus those unable to carry a fetus to full term. Subfertility is a broader term, indicating couples who are less fertile than would be considered "normal." Primary infertility refers to those who have never had a child; another definition of primary infertility is those who have conceived a child but cannot carry to term. Secondary infertility refers to those who have at least one living child but are having difficulty conceiving another.

INFORMED CONSENT A process that lets the patient know the risks and benefits of a medical or research procedure. Mandated by federal regulations in the United States, informed consent forms are required before patients enter into research studies or have invasive procedures performed. Informed consent forms tell the patient about the risks and benefits of the procedure or study, and confirm the voluntary nature of participation.

INTRACYTOPLASMIC SPERM INJECTION (ICSI) A relatively new procedure (of a category sometimes called micromanipulation) where a single sperm is injected directly into the egg. Can enable fertilization in cases of very low sperm count or abnormal sperm.

INTRAUTERINE INSEMINATION (IUI) A procedure in which sperm (from either the woman's partner or a donor) are washed and prepared, and inserted into her cervix through a very thin tube at the time of ovulation. Useful in the case of hostile cervical mucus, poor sperm-mucus interaction, or other problems.

IN VITRO FERTILIZATION (IVF) The first ART procedure. Following superovulation using medications under an infertility specialist's careful observation, eggs are aspirated (extracted with a very fine needle) from a woman's ovaries. In a sterile and carefully controlled laboratory environment, the eggs are fertilized with washed and prepared sperm. The zygotes that develop are transferred into the woman's uterus. In vitro also refers to anything done in glass, in a test tube, or in a laboratory. Studies may refer to "in vitro" results meaning results seen on a more basic (e.g., cellular) level. ("In vivo" refers to results seen in a living organism.)

-ITIS A suffix attached to the name of organs to indicate infection or inflammation. For instance, epididymitis is an inflammation of the epididymis.

KALLMANN'S SYNDROME A very rare disorder in which the hypothalamus does not release any GnRH.

KARYOTYPING To see if there are genetic anomalies present, a picture of the genetic makeup of a person or animal is constructed by showing cells in descending order of size.

LAPAROSCOPY Examination of the pelvic region by using a laparoscope, a small fiberoptic device that is inserted into the abdomen to either diagnose or correct fertility or other problems.

LAPAROTOMY Surgical procedure in which an incision is made in the abdomen.

LH SURGE The surge of LH that signals ovulation to take place. See also Luteinizing Hormone.

LUTEAL PHASE *See Basal Body Temperature (BBT).*

LUTEAL PHASE DEFECT When, in the second half of the menstrual cycle, a woman does not produce enough progesterone to prepare the uterine lining for an embryo's implantation. Usually diagnosed with an endometrial biopsy.

LUTEINIZED UNRUPTURED FOLLICLES When eggs are properly prepared for ovulation but not released; may happen occasionally or as a syndrome.

LUTEINIZING HORMONE (LH) A hormone released by the pituitary under the direction of the hypothalamus that stimulates reproductive hormonal function in males and females. In males, LH is necessary for sperm and testosterone production. In females, LH is necessary for ovulation and the menstrual cycle. When estrogen levels from the secretory phase of the menstrual cycle reach a zenith, an LH surge occurs; approximately 24 hours after this surge, the egg is released from the follicle.

MENORRHAGIA Excessive menstrual flow marked by too many days of flow, too heavy a flow, or both.

METRORRHAGIA Bleeding from the uterus at any time other than during menstruation.

MISCARRIAGE *See Abortion.*

MITTLESCHMERZ Discomfort some women feel in the pelvic region with ovulation.

MOLAR PREGNANCY (ALSO KNOWN AS HYDATID MOLE) A very rare degenerative disorder where the chorionic villi turn into multiple bubble-like cysts. The uterus expands and can hemorrhage. Can be very dangerous to the mother. Sometimes diagnosed by excessively increasing hCG levels.

MONOPHASIC *See Basal Body Temperature (BBT).*

MOTILITY Ability to move.

NEURAL TUBE DEFECTS A congenital anomaly in which the spinal column or other nervous system structures do not develop properly during early embryonic growth.

OLIGOMENORRHEA Irregular or infrequent menstrual periods. Can also refer to scanty (light) menstrual periods.

OLIGOSPERMIA Semen that does not contain sufficient numbers of sperm; actual values will differ based on lab normal ranges used and physician interpretation.

OOCYTE The very young egg, in the ovary, before it has matured.

OVARIAN CYST A round, generally fluid-filled, sac in the ovary.

OVIDUCTS *See Fallopian Tubes.*

OVULATION When a follicle in the ovary releases an egg.

OVULATION INDUCTION When medical treatments are used to stimulate ovulation.

OVUM Another word for egg.

OXYTOCIN A hormone secreted by the pituitary that causes the uterus to contract; also causes the release of breast milk. May be given as a drug to induce labor or facilitate contraction of the uterus after labor (also known by its trade name, Pitocin).

PATENT When a tube or organ is open or passable.

PELVIC INFLAMMATORY DISEASE (PID) Infection of the pelvic organs that may be ascending (in the case of STIs, and most common reference) or descending (in the case of expansion of infection from another cause—like appendicitis—to the pelvic organs). Can cause acute illness as well as infertility from scarring and adhesions. Treatment is generally with antibiotics, often administered intravenously at first.

PITUITARY GLAND Sitting right beneath the hypothalamus in the brain, the pituitary exerts hormonal control over many systems in the body, including the reproductive system.

PLACENTA Soft, round, blood-enriched tissues that develop with the infant to allow maternal blood supply to nourish the growing embryo and fetus. It allows oxygen and nutrition to be delivered to the infant, and takes waste products from the infant to be eliminated by the mother's system. Also secretes estrogen and progesterone to help maintain a proper hormonal environment throughout pregnancy. Problems with the placenta can cause fetal injury, pre-term labor, and stillbirth. Weighing about one pound at full term, the placenta is delivered as the "afterbirth."

POLAR BODY During meiosis of a woman's ovum, the unnecessary 23 chromosomes are discarded in the form of a polar body.

POLYCYSTIC OVARY SYNDROME (ALSO KNOWN AS PCO, PCOS, OR STEIN LEVENTHAL SYNDROME) A condition in which follicles in ovaries are inundated with too much LH, causing cyst formation within ovaries and secretion (in response to the excess LH) of androgens. Symptoms may include excess hair growth, infertility, or weight gain, although some women with PCO are asymptomatic.

POST-COITAL TEST (ALSO KNOWN AS PCT OR HUHNERS' TEST) A test to assess how well sperm penetrate the cervical mucus. The number of healthy sperm present in a woman's cervix are measured microscopically after intercourse. Can reveal the presence of hostile mucus. Some researchers question this test, however, indicating that there are cases of women with negative PCT who had sperm present in their fallopian tubes.

PRIMARY INFERTILITY *See Infertility.*

PROGESTERONE Hormone released by the corpus luteum after ovulation. See also Corpus Luteum, BBT monitoring, and hCG.

PROGESTERONE WITHDRAWAL A diagnostic procedure used to assess irregularity in the menstrual cycle; indicates if hormones are working correctly to manage the cycle.

PROLACTIN Hormone released by the pituitary gland that governs milk production.

PROLIFERATIVE PHASE *See Basal Body Temperature (BBT).*

PROSTATE GLAND This male reproductive organ contributes an alkaline prostatic fluid to the semen, which allows liquefaction of the semen once entering the cervix.

PROSTATITIS Inflammation or infection of the prostate gland, may result in damage to sperm.

REPRODUCTIVE ENDOCRINOLOGY The study of the endocrinology of reproduction, often with an emphasis on infertility.

RETROVERTED UTERUS Backward tilting uterus, where the uterus leans toward the back.

SALPINGECTOMY Surgical removal of a fallopian tube in part or whole.

SALPINGITIS Inflammation of the fallopian tube. Some physicians use this term and PID interchangeably.

SALPINGOSTOMY Surgically opening the fallopian tubes; may be performed during a laparoscopy or a laparotomy.

SCROTUM The double pouch of skin in the male, beneath the penis, that contains the testicles and part of the spermatic cord.

SECONDARY INFERTILITY *See Infertility.*

SECONDARY SEX CHARACTERISTICS Characteristics of sexual maturation other than menstrual cycle in the woman or sperm development and delivery in the male; under the direction of the endocrine system. Examples include breast development in women, voice changing in men, and pubic hair growth in men and women.

SECRETORY PHASE *See Basal Body Temperature (BBT).*

SEMEN The fluid that is released during ejaculation. Composed of secretions from the seminal vesicles, prostate gland, and several other glands in the male reproductive tract, in addition to sperm.

SEMEN ANALYSIS Following abstinence for (usually) two or three days, a semen sample is analyzed in a laboratory. The test assesses sperm quantity, concentration, morphology (shape of sperm), and motility (movement of sperm). Analysis also checks for presence of white blood cells, immature sperm, sperm agglutination (clumping), pH composition of semen, and other characteristics.

SEMINAL VESICLES Lying behind the male's bladder, these vesicles produce much of the semen volume, as well as the sugar in the semen, which provides nourishment and energy for the sperm.

SEXUALLY TRANSMITTED INFECTIONS (STI) Infections transmitted sexually. There are many types, but some of the major ones are chlamydia, gonorrhea, syphilis, chancroid, ureaplasma (mycoplasma), herpes simplex virus type II, human papilloma virus (causes genital warts, cervical cancer), human immunodeficiency virus (HIV, the virus that causes AIDS), and hepatitis B. May also be called sexually transmitted diseases (STD) or venereal diseases (VD).

SONOGRAM *See Ultrasound.*

SPERM (ALSO KNOWN AS SPERMATOZOA) Refers to male genetic-information-carrying sex cell.

SPERM COUNT The quantity of sperm in an ejaculate.

SPERM MATURATION The process by which sperm mature and learn to swim. Sperm take about 90 days to reach maturity, as they progress through the male's reproductive system.

SPERM MORPHOLOGY Shape of sperm.

SPERM MOTILITY Swimming and movement ability of sperm.

SPERM WASHING A technique to prepare sperm for insertion into a woman's reproductive system. In normal reproduction, sperm are prepared—capacitated—when they pass through cervical mucus into the uterus. When sperm (in semen) are inserted directly into the uterus without going through the cervical mucus they are not properly prepared, and the semen is toxic to both the sperm and the uterus. Unprepared sperm are not able to swim to and fertilize the egg. To prevent this harmful response when performing intrauterine insemination and ARTs, the sperm are prepared with a laboratory process called sperm washing. This process allows the sperm to be in the same state they would have been in had they passed through the cervical mucus. When the sperm are inserted into the woman's uterus, they are appropriately readied and able to seek out and fertilize the egg.

SPERMATOCELE A cyst within the epididymis that contains sperm. May be small or large, requiring no treatment, observation, or surgical repair.

SPERMATOCYTE The very young sperm, before it has matured.

SPERMATOGENESIS The process of sperm production and maturation in the testicles.

SPINNBARKEIT *See Cervical Mucus.*

STERILITY A condition that prevents reproductive function in either males or females. May be natural, due to illness or surgery, or elected as a form of surgical contraception. Also means free of living organisms, such as in the case of "a sterile environment."

STILLBIRTH When a fetus dies after 20 weeks of gestation, but prior to delivery.

SUBFERTILITY *See Infertility.*

SUPEROVULATION (ALSO KNOWN AS CONTROLLED OVARIAN HYPER-STIMULATION) Use of fertility medications to induce ovulation of many eggs. May be used with ARTs or alone.

TERATOGENIC Causes or contributes to abnormal development of embryo.

TESTICULAR STRESS PATTERN May refer to semen analysis in which there is depression of sperm production (low count), abnormal motility (movement), and/or abnormal morphology (shape). Can occur transiently, due to illness, varicocele, injury, or elevated scrotal temperature.

TESTOSTERONE The hormone responsible for secondary sex characteristics and sperm development in males, testosterone is released under the control of the endocrine system.

TOCOLYSIS Stoppage of uterine contractions. Tocolytic medications halt uterine contractions.

TORSION The twisting of an organ. Can be very serious. Some organs that can suffer from torsion: testicles, ovaries, fallopian tubes, and organs related to digestion.

TUBAL LIGATION Surgical contraceptive procedure in the woman in which the fallopian tubes are severed or tied under anesthesia to prevent conception.

ULTRASOUND Used frequently in infertility evaluation to assess follicle development, ovary health, etc.; also used in pregnancy evaluation to assess fetal growth and development, and health status. Uses high-frequency sound waves to create an image of internal tissues without the danger of x-rays or radiation. May be transvaginal (with a wand shaped device that is inserted into the vagina) or transabdominal (with a round device that is circulated on the abdomen).

UROLOGY The medical specialty concentrating on urinary tracts of men and women and the genital tracts of men.

UTERINE FIBROID (ALSO KNOWN AS FIBROMA) A benign tumor found in the uterus.

UTERUS The muscular organ in a woman's pelvic region that carries and nourishes a growing baby.

VARICOCELE Dilation of one or more of the veins that carry blood in the scrotum; essentially varicose veins of the scrotal area. May be a cause of male infertility as a result of elevated scrotal temperatures, which are detrimental to sperm development and function. Some studies question the relationship between varicocele and male factor infertility.

VARICOCELECTOMY Surgical procedure in which varicoceles are removed.

VAS DEFERENS One of the tubes sperm pass through en route from the testicles toward the seminal vesicles and prostate gland.

VASECTOMY Surgical contraceptive procedure in the man in which the vas deferens are severed or tied under anesthesia to prevent conception.

VENEREAL DISEASE *See Sexually Transmitted Infections.*

VIABLE Able to live alone; for instance, the stage at which a fetus is able to live on its own outside the mother's uterus.

ZYGOTE The result of the sperm-egg union; a fertilized egg.

ZYGOTE INTRAFALLOPIAN TRANSFER (ZIFT) An ART procedure that evolved from the IVF and GIFT procedures. Following superovulation using medications under an infertility specialist's careful observation, eggs are aspirated (extracted with a very fine needle) from a woman's ovaries. In a sterile and carefully controlled laboratory environment, the eggs are fertilized with washed and prepared sperm. The zygotes that develop are transferred into the woman's fallopian tubes. This modification of traditional IVF and GIFT is thought to have higher success rates in some women than its predecessors, due to the placement of the zygotes in the fallopian tubes rather than the uterus, and due to the placement of a zygote rather than unfertilized eggs and sperm.

References and Resources

Organizations

American Board of Obstetrics and Gynecology
2915 Vine Street, Suite 300
Dallas, Texas 75204
(214) 871-1619
fax: (214) 871-1943

The American College of Obstetricians and Gynecologists
409 12th Street SW
PO Box 96920
Washington, D.C. 20090-6920

American Medical Association
1101 Vermont Avenue NW
Washington, D.C. 20005
(202) 789-7400

American Society for Reproductive Medicine
1209 Montgomery Highway
Birmingham, Alabama 35216-2809
(205) 978-5000
fax: (205) 978-5005

Centers for Disease Control and Prevention

1600 Clifton Road NE

Atlanta, Georgia 30333

(404) 639-3311

InterNational Council on Infertility Information Dissemination (INCIID)

PO Box 6836

Arlington, Virginia 22206

(703) 379-9178

fax: (703) 379-1593

National Center for Health Statistics

6525 Belcrest Road

Hyattsville, Maryland 20782

nchsquery@cdc.gov

(301) 436-8500

National Institutes of Health (NIH)

9000 Rockville Pike

Bethesda, Maryland 20892

RESOLVE, Inc.

1310 Broadway

Somerville, Massachusetts 02144-1779

Business office: (617) 623-1156

National HelpLine: (617) 623-0744

fax: (617) 623-0252

World Organization of the Ovulation Method/Billings

Billings Family Life Centre

27, Alexandra Parade Fitzroy North
Victoria 3068 Australia
(03) 9481-1722

Notable Web Sites

American Board of Obstetrics and Gynecology www.abog.org

American College of Obstetricians and Gynecologists www.acog.com

American Medical Association www.ama-assn.org

Atlanta Reproductive Health Center www.ivf.com

American Society for Reproductive Medicine www.asrm.org

Centers for Disease Control and Prevention www.cdc.gov

InterNational Council on Infertility Information Dissemination (INCIID)
www.inciid.org

MD Consult (excellent online resource; comprehensive personalized
searches for journal articles, guidelines, and entire medical textbooks)
www.mdconsult.com

National Center for Health Statistics www.cdc.gov/nchswww

National Institute of Child Health and Human Development
www.nih.gov/nichd/home.html

National Institutes of Health (NIH) www.nih.gov

New York On Line Access to Health www.noah.cuny.edu

OVID (excellent online resource, journals, etc.) gateway.ovid.com

World Health Organization www.who.int

World Organization of the Ovulation Method/Billings www.billings-centre.ab.ca

Books

American Medical Women's Association Guide to Fertility and Reproductive Health, The by Payne R., Stewart S., Dell Books

Before You Conceive: The Complete Prepregnancy Guide by Sussman J.R., Levitt B., Bantam Doubleday Dell

Conceptions & Misconceptions: A Guide Through the Maze of in Vitro Fertilization & Other Assisted Reproduction Techniques by Meldrum D.R., Wisot A.L., Hartley and Marks Press

Couple's Guide to Fertility: Updated with the Newest Scientific Techniques to Help You Have a Baby, The by Goldstein M., Fuerst M., Berger G.S., Main Street Books

Getting Pregnant! by Frisch M.J., Rapoport G., H.P. Books

Getting Pregnant and Staying Pregnant: Overcoming Infertility and Managing Your High-Risk Pregnancy by Raab D., Hunter House Books

Getting Pregnant: What Couples Need to Know Right Now by Lauersen N.H., Bouchez C., Fawcett Books

Getting Pregnant When You Thought You Couldn't: The Interactive Guide That Helps You Up the Odds by Rosenberg H.S., Epstein Y.M., Sandler B., Warner Books

How to Be a Successful Fertility Patient: Your Guide to Getting the Best Possible Medical Help to Have a Baby by Robin P., Quill Books

How to Get Pregnant: With the New Technology by Silber S.J., Warner Books

How to Prevent Miscarriage and Other Crises of Pregnancy by Semchyshyn S., Colman C., Macmillan

In Pursuit of Fertility: A Fertility Expert Tells You How to Get Pregnant by Franklin R.R., Buttram V.C., Brockman D.K., Henry Holt

In Vitro Fertilization: The A.R.T. of Making Babies by Sher G., Davis V.M., Stoess J., Facts on File

Infertility: A Practical Guide for the Physician by Hammond M.G., Talbot L.M., Blackwell Scientific Publications

Pregnancy Journal, *The* by Harris A.C., Chronicle Books

Preventing Miscarriage: The Good News by Scher J., Dix C., HarperCollins

Taber's Cyclopedic Medical Dictionary Rice K.M., F.A. Davis Company

Taking Charge of Infertility by Johnston P.I., Perspectives Press

Taking Charge of Your Fertility: The Definitive Guide to Natural Birth Control and Pregnancy Achievement by Weschler T., Harperperennial Library

World Health Organization Manual for the Standardized Investigation of the Infertile Couple, by Rowe P.J., Comhaire F.H., Hargreave T.B., Mellows H.J., World Health Organization, Cambridge University Press

You Can Have a Baby by Bellina J., Wilson J., Crown Publishers

Your Fertility Signals: Using Them to Achieve or Avoid Pregnancy Naturally, by Winstein M., Smooth Stone Press

Medical Textbooks

Benson and Pernoll's Handbook of Obstetrics and Gynecology (Ninth Edition) by Benson R.C. and Pernoll M.L., McGraw-Hill, Inc.

Clinical Gynecologic Endocrinology and Infertility by Speroff L, Glass RH, Kase, NG, Lippincott-Raven

Danforth's Handbook of Obstetrics and Gynecology by Scott J.R., Disaia P.J., Hammond C.B., Lippincott-Raven

Kistner's Gynecology: Princples and Practice (Sixth Edition) by Kistner R.W., Mosby Year Book, Inc.

Textbook of Reproductive Medicine (Second Edition) by Carr B.R., Blackwell R.E., Appleton and Lange

Williams Obstetrics (Twentieth Edition) by Cunningham F.G., MacDonald P.C., Gant N.F., et al, Appleton and Lange

Medical Journals

American Journal of Obstetrics and Gynecology

Clinical Obstetrics and Gynecology

Human Reproduction

International Journal of Fertility

Journal of the American Medical Association

Journal of Fertility and Sterility, The

Journal of Reproductive Medicine

Medical Clinics of North America

Mortality and Morbidity Weekly Report (a CDC publication)

New England Journal of Medicine

Obstetrical Clinics of North America

Obstetrics and Gynecology

Index